Praise from Pro

"This book is a treasure I wish I had when I started my practice. Victoria takes the complex subject of weight loss and breaks it down into an easy, well thought out, and manageable system that ensures long lasting results. Everything you need to be successful with your weight loss clients is in this. The result: the guesswork for weight loss hypnosis is gone and a beautiful, compassionate program is delivered. Bravo, Victoria!"

Stephanie Conkle, Clinical Hypnotherapist
Creator of the Profound Somnambulism Protocol
www.StephanieConkle.com

"I recommend Victoria's book, as it outlines a 3-month protocol for hypnotists to help clients reach their individual power. The results are lasting multi-faceted changes to peoples' bodies, thought processes, and their lives. Now there is a process to build change slowly and in digestible measures, using cross-sections of techniques through live sessions and subsequent recordings and homework. What a great addition to your library and practice."

Cheryl J Elman, CH, CI, CMT, BS Ed
www.DaveElmanHypnosisInstitute.com

"Victoria Gallagher provides a real-world, tested, and powerful resource to the hypnosis field. This book goes beyond scripts and is a comprehensive manual with phenomenal methods to benefit both new and seasoned hypnotists. If you want to WORK SMART in your hypnosis sessions, this book will make you a more effective weight loss hypnotist."

Jason Linett
Host of the Work Smart Hypnosis Podcast
https://WorkSmartHypnosis.com

"This book is more than scripts. It is a solid weight loss program designed to benefit hypnotists' clients and help hypnotists build an amazing practice."

Helena Jehnichen
Certified Clinical Hypnotherapist
www.FlourishHypnosis.com

"This book is full of rock solid, fundamental strategies to help a person lose any amount of weight. The techniques and strategies are sound and thoughtful; the content well-articulated to help millions of people worldwide face a pressing problem."

Scott Sandland, C.Ht.
Founder of Hypnosis Practitioner Training Institute
https://HypnosisTrainingInstitute.org/

"I love Victoria Gallagher's approach to weight loss. Her extensive knowledge of hypnotherapy, coupled with her in-depth understanding of the world of diet and exercise, puts this book ULTIMATE WEIGHT LOSS POWER well ahead of other script books."

Dr. Tracy Riley, LCSW
www.TracyRiley.com

"This book delivers a well-crafted 12-week protocol that sets the path for lasting weight loss success. Taking you from laying the foundation and eliminating limiting beliefs to facilitating the development of healthy life-long habits and beyond, Victoria leaves no stone unturned. Whether you are looking for a fresh perspective and new tools to add to your toolbox, Victoria provides this...and more."

Kerrilee Pietroski
Board Certified Hypnotherapist and Eating Psychology Coach
www.KPEmpoweringU.com

"Don't let the name fool you. Victoria Gallagher's Ultimate Weight Loss Power Hypnotherapy Script Book is much more than what the title suggests. Victoria has produced a complete weight loss program for any practicing Consulting Hypnotist or Hypnotherapist. Even seasoned practitioners will benefit handsomely with this program. Once again, Victoria delivers as a true professional."

Tom Nicoli, BCH, CI, CPC
Board Certified Hypnotist & Personal Development Coach
www.ProsperUSA.com

"Scripts, hypnotherapy training techniques, and a week by week, easy to replicate breakdown offers the essential components for an effective weight loss program for any hypnotherapist. This book has it all!"

Taressa Riazzi, Certified Hypnotherapist
www.TaressaRiazzi.com

"Even with 30 plus years of experience, I find this book to be a wonderful tool for my practice. Hypnotherapists can help their clients discover healthy habits and slim, trim bodies, and this resource will help. I can't wait to get started using it with my clients!"

Tracy Bonczyk
Board Certified Hypnotherapist, Instructor, Reiki Master
www.HypnosisCareSolutions.com

"In this easy to read and captivating book, Victoria combines personal accounts with years of professional experiences working with weight loss clients. Regardless of if you're a hypnotist or someone desiring weight loss, this easy to follow program will lead you to weight loss, while developing a lifestyle to prevent the problem from returning. My only problem with this book is that I did not write it. As for you, get it TODAY!"

Dr. Will Horton
Psychologist and author of "Habits for Success"
www.AASolved.com

"Victoria Gallagher's 'Ultimate Weight Loss Power Hypnotherapy Script Book' is the definitive guide for practitioners looking to help their clients with the critical issue of weight loss. The information is comprehensive and offers a well-organized layout. In time, Victoria's writing will prove to be the standard for weight loss."

Selena D. Valentine
Founder of HypnoBiz Media and Certified Hypnotist/Instructor
www.HypnoBiz.com

"This book is brilliant. It provides a comprehensive and powerful weight loss and management program designed for hypnotherapists to deliver results to their clients. Victoria's approach is practical and realistic, covering everything from creating a niche in weight management to getting clients to commit to change. The superb framework of this content includes scripts, tools, homework assignments, and practical advice to get your client engaged and motivated. This is an amazing and much needed contribution to the hypnosis world."

Kaz Riley, BSc PDHyp PHyp BSCH NLPPA
Clinical Hypnotist
http://KazRiley.com

"I sure wish this book was available to me twenty-three years ago when I was creating my weight loss program. It would have benefitted me and my weight loss hypnosis clients. This is the book I had always wanted to write...and now I don't have to. Victoria masterfully details, step-by-step, how to structure and conduct weight loss sessions for hypnotherapy clients (and yourself)."

Roger Moore
Medical Hypnotherapist
www.HypnosisHealthInfo.com

"I wish I would have had this book when I started my hypnotherapy practice. Victoria's script book covers everything you need to know to help you get your weight loss hypnosis business off the ground. For beginners, reading Ultimate Weight Loss Power is an exceptional way to equip yourself with tried and true techniques. For advanced hypnotherapists, this is a refresher worth diving into."

Joi Stevens, Certified Hypnotherapist
www.BelieveInHypnotherapy.com

"This is a book for newbies and seasoned professionals who are on the hunt for a highly effective weekly weight loss program for their practice. Victoria offers highly effective inductions, resources for royalty free music, weight loss scripts, and her S.M.A.R.T. Goals Systems. Take advantage of Victoria's 20 plus years as a leader/visionary in the hypnosis field and make this into your own."

Jackie Fokkens (CHT)
Personal Coach and Hypnotist - St. Louis, Missouri
www.PersonalCoachingByJackie.com

"This book offers new and seasoned hypnotherapists all the tools needed to help their clients achieve weight loss. Victoria offers step-by-step guidance that has been researched and proven effective for multitudes of people. With 1/3 of Americans classified as obese, this means hypnotherapists have access to a market of more than 100 million potential clients. If you do not already have a thriving weight loss business, this book can help you achieve one. I cannot recommend this book enough! All power to you and those whose lives you will improve with this wonderful program."

Freddy Jacquin, BSc (Hons) Clinical Hypnosis
https://FreddyJacquin.com/

"This book is a wonderful resource for a hypnotist's interested in weight loss programs. Victoria takes you through every aspect of the process, beginning to end, business-wise and client focused. You will learn how to create a systematic approach, based on a foundational system that builds step-by-step. Gain insights on how to structure pricing sessions, as well as how to teach your clients to take responsibility for their change. Victoria is the go-to expert on this subject."

Amber Rose Cox, BCH
www.MaineHypnosisCenter.com

"Buy this book! It's a detailed and comprehensive tool, revealing a different approach to weight loss to the novice or experienced hypnotherapist. This 12-week program includes education and scripts that address foundational beliefs, hunger, visualizing, accessing the cause, drinking water, exercising, eating healthy, metabolism, banishing old patterns, melting fat, reshaping the body, and maintenance. It's wonderful and necessary information!"

Jennifer Kane, DC, FIAMA, CPT, CH
www.DrJenniferKane.com

"Victoria's years of research and depth of understanding show in this book. It is a useful collection of scripts that every practitioner in this area should have access to. Well done!"

Michael Watson CHt
Director, Phoenix Services for Personal Development
www.Phoenix-Services.org

"I've been looking for a program to use in my practice and now I have found it. Victoria Gallagher's Ultimate Weight Loss Hypnotherapy Script Book provides a comprehensive system with well-constructed scripts and specific goals to guide the client to success from start to finish."

Joni Neidigh
Psychotherapist, Hypnotherapist
Jonineidighhypnosis.com

"This is undoubtedly the best and most useful book I have ever read on the subject of weight loss. It is inspirational and clearly written by someone who understands the struggle with weight loss. Victoria has 'been there, done that, and worn the T-shirt' and I believe there is no substitute for life experience. Everything happens for a reason. The program in the book is complete—a 12-week program ready to go! It's full of little gems and nuggets I intend to use in my own private practice."

David J Birch
Clinical Hypnotherapist & HypnoPsychotherapist Ireland
www.HypnoBandKildare.com

"As a hypnosis educator and trainer for over 20 years, this book is at the top of my reading list suggestions for students. The book is simple for the new hypnotist, yet inclusive of techniques that even seasoned hypnotists can draw upon. Victoria's ability to write and instruct is amazing. Content is easily understood and flowing. A true diamond for practitioners and self-hypnosis enthusiasts alike."

Sandra Bemis
Board Certified Hypnotist Certified Instructor
www.SandraBemis.com

"I have worked as a Certified Clinical Hypnotherapist for 15 years and this book is one of the best I've read for weight management. It is clear and concise, addressing all the important areas in an efficient manner. This approach is highly recommended for hypnotherapists who are serious about helping their clients release weight. The program has everything you need, from A to Z. Victoria, thank you for sharing your approach with us!"

Pierre Benoit, RCCH
Registered Counseling Clinical Hypnotherapist
www.HypnotherapyMontreal.com

"Victoria Gallagher has written a thorough quick start guide for any hypnotist wanting to help their clients with weight loss. I've been doing this work for over 35 years and now consider this book a must-read because it is practical and takes you step-by-step through the process."

Lisa Kunschick
Certified Master Hypnotist, Stage Hypnotist
www.UpYourCupSize.com

"Victoria has formulated a holistic, complete approach to weight loss. Her program thoroughly addresses every aspect of weight loss with care and love, while creating a supportive space for both the practitioner and the client to succeed and thrive."

Miri Malkin
Clinical Hypnotherapist
www.MiriMalkin.com

"Well done, Victoria! This book is filled with fantastic tips and an easy to follow model to resolve core issues associated with weight. The hard work of structuring a comprehensive weight-loss protocol has already been done for you in this book."

Dr. Steve G. Jones
Ed.D. Clinical Hypnotherapist
www.SteveGJones.com

"This book walks you through weight loss & stepping into your best you through hypnosis. Victoria has generously included forms and questionnaires, as well as induction, hypnotherapy scripts skillfully crafted to assist your client to lose weight and enhance the mind and body."

Sharron Magyar
Golden Heart Hypnosis, Golden Heart School of Hypnosis
www.SharronMagyar.com

"Victoria's knowledge and experience are wonderfully captured in this book. The way it's structured insures you will have all the resources you need to create a winning program for your clients, and therefore, you."

Mr. Turan Mirza, Hypnotist, Speaker, Trainer
Northern Ireland
www.Feel-Good.today

"ULTIMATE WEIGHT LOSS POWER HYPNOTHERAPY SCRIPT BOOK is fantastic! I'm looking forward to sharing this program with my clients who are seeking weight loss through hypnotherapy. They can finally release their weight and feel fantastic in their bodies! Thank you, Victoria!"

Bessie Estonactoc
Hypnotherapist & Change Maker Mentor
www.WishHawaii.com

"This book is golden, an impressive well written guide that is both comprehensive and easy to implement. Victoria's valuable insight and recommendations are from years of personal experience formulated with truly heartfelt and sincere inspiration which resonates on every page, every word. This is the start to helping clients achieve weight loss success, which will translate into referrals and hypnotist success. Powerful!

Lori Ann Redlinski, CH
Advance Health Hypnosis
www.AdvanceHealthHypnosis.com

"The Ultimate Weight Loss Power Pack Script book is "the book" for anyone working with weight loss clients. Victoria lays out the road map for practitioners, step-by-step, session by session. This is a must have book to help your clients achieve their goals."

Toni Macri Reiner
Clinical Hypnotist
www.IndianaHypnosisforChange.com

"This is the perfect business in a box, or should I say business in a book, for any hypnotherapist, new or experienced, who wants to work with weight issues. The book is a wealth of knowledge and the total experience is eye opening. The scripts are easily adapted for your own personal style."

Bruce Bonczyk, CHt
Hypnosis instructor, Reiki Master
http://SouthernCaliforniaStopSmokingCenter.com

"I am drawn to how simple and easy Victoria's model is to follow. The use of hypnosis with a client centered approach to find the core issues of weight struggles is effective, leading to the formation of long lasting new good habits. I am very grateful to have discovered and read the book. It'll be put to good use in my practice."

Cristina Balhui
Emotional Intelligence Coach
https://www.IntegratedHolisticTherapies.com

"This book is fantastic! It's a well thought out and detailed protocol, ideal for hypnotists of all levels. Make it a must-read if you wish to implement a powerful weight management program into your practice."

Shana Rosenthal, Certified Hypnotist
www.ShanaHypnotist.com

"This is the ultimate weight loss/script book!!! It offers insights to weight loss by addressing the many aspects of healing, reflection, release, expanded awareness, and tools for a lifetime. The process unfolds like an adventure in wellness. Loving this book and will make great use of this fantastic program."

Valerie James, CHt
Clinical/Transpersonal Hypnotherapist, Certified Brain Health Coach
www.BloomingMindWorks.com

"I absolutely recommend this. Victoria's genuine desire to contribute to society in positive, winning ways, is evidenced throughout this book and its contents. It offers a masterful blend and simplicity at the same time. The scripts are masterful and the step-by-step instructions are easy to follow. This book is valuable to hypnotists who want to create a successful weight loss business, and even to individuals with a strong desire to work on their own weight loss goals. It's a WIN-WIN."

Phil WIN-
IHypnosis Trainer/ Results Focus Coach
www.WinningWays.info

ULTIMATE WEIGHT LOSS POWER

Hypnotherapy Script Book

ULTIMATE WEIGHT LOSS POWER

Hypnotherapy Script Book

12-Week Hypnosis Program For Hypnotherapists

Victoria M. Gallagher

Copyright © 2019 by Victoria M. Gallagher

Cover and Illustrations by Michelle Casal

All rights reserved. This book or any portion thereof may not be reproduced or used in any manner whatsoever without the express written permission of the publisher except for the use of brief quotations in a book review.

You have permission to use these scripts to make private recordings for your clients. You may not publish these scripts or sell them in written form.

For more hypnosis scripts go to www.hyptalk.com

Printed in the United States of America

First Printing, 2019

ISBN 9781678749583

Independently Published

www.VictoriaMGallagher.com

Table of Contents

PRAISE FROM PROFESSIONAL HYPNOTISTS I
FOREWORD XXIII
INTRODUCTION 1
   Who Am I? 1
   Why is this Program Different? 3
   Who are You? 5
   Setting the Appointment 6
   How to Price Your Service 7
   Hypnotic Recordings 11
   Background Music 12
   Program Outline 12
      Week 1: The Foundation 12
      Week 2: Hunger Dial 13
      Week 3: Screen of the Mind 13
      Week 4: Access the Cause 13
      Week 5: Drinking Water 13
      Week 6: Exercise 13
      Week 7: Eat Healthy 13
      Week 8: Metabolism 14
      Week 9: Banish Old Patterns of Behavior for Good 14
      Week 10: Melt Fat 14
      Week 11: Reshape Your Body 14
      Week 12: Maintenance 14
   Assigning Homework 15
WEEK 1: FOUNDATION 17
   Step One: Set a Smart Goal 18
      Definition of a Goal 18
      "Pink Bunny" 19
      Be Specific 20
      Money Analogy 20
      Sports Analogy 21

Step Two: Progressive Muscle Relaxation and Negative Beliefs 24
- Pre-Talk 24
- What is Progressive Muscle Relaxation? 25
- Progressive Muscle Relaxation 28

Negative Beliefs Script 33
- Trance termination 36

Step Three: Create Powerful Positive Affirmations: 37
- How to Convert Negative Beliefs into Positive Powerful Affirmations? 37
- Create an Affirmation Poster 40

WEEK 2: HUNGER SCALE 43
- Education about the Hunger Scale 43
- Hunger Scale Script 44

WEEK 3: VISUALIZATION 49
- Education about Visualization 49
- Screen of the Mind Script 50

WEEK 4: ACCESS THE CAUSE 55
- Education about Regression 55
- Access the Cause Script 56

WEEK 5: DRINK WATER 61
- Education about Drinking Water 61
- Drink Water Script: 62

WEEK 6: EXERCISE 69
- Education about Exercise 69
- Exercise Script 70

WEEK 7: EAT HEALTHY 75
- Education about Healthy Eating: 75
- Eat Healthy Script 76

WEEK 8: METABOLISM 81
- Education about Metabolism 81
- Metabolism Script 82

WEEK 9: BANISH OLD PATTERNS OF BEHAVIOR FOR GOOD 89
- Education About Swish 89
- Swish Script 91

WEEK 10: MELT FAT 95
- Education about Melting Fat 95
- Melt Fat Script 96

WEEK 11: RESHAPE YOUR BODY 101
    Education about Reshaping Your Body 101
    Reshape Your Body Script 102

WEEK 12: MAINTENANCE 107
    Education about Maintenance 107
    Maintenance Script 107

FORMS 111
    Client Agreement 113
    Policies 115
    S.M.A.R.T. Goal System Worksheet 117
    Weight Loss Questionnaire 118

HAND-OUTS 121
    Week 1: Create an Affirmation Poster 123
    Week 1: Weight Affirmations 124
    Week 2: Hunger Scale Diagram 126
    Week 2: Emotional Eating Journal 127
    Week 3: About Visualization 128
    Week 5: Water 129
    Week 5: Water Drinking Weekly Journal 131
    Week 6: How to Get Back into the Exercise Habit 132
    Week 6: Simple Exercise Journal 135
    Week 7: Nutrition 136
    Week 7: Healthy Eating Plan 138

INDUCTION SCRIPTS 139
    Walking Through a Desert 141
    Down the Stairs 145
    Healing Light 147
    Healthy Body 149
    My Elman 153
    Progressive Muscle Relaxation 156

TRANCE TERMINATION SCRIPTS 161
    Drift off or Wake up 163
    Waking on the Count of 5 164

FINAL THOUGHTS 165

ABOUT THE AUTHOR 167

Foreword

I was always the skinny guy, never struggling with my weight. Then I hit 40, and as magically predicted, all the weight I should have gained from my Standard American Diet (S.A.D.) showed up in a single year. As a professional hypnotist, I used my main tool, hypnosis, to help me change my eating patterns, commit to increasing my physical activity, and make changes I felt were necessary.

It worked. Well, until I had two years of major foot surgeries in my mid-40s. I wore a boot and rode a knee-scooter for almost a year, making me mostly no weight bearing. During those years the pounds piled on again, to the point I was 40-50 pounds overweight. It wasn't just the physical limitations that lent to my situation; it was the depression and anxiety around some permeant limitations that drove me to find comfort in my old S.A.D. eating patterns.

As a professional hypnotist, being overweight is not a great selling point for your services. So, I lost the weight again. To do this, I used techniques Victoria reveals in this book.

Now I am in my mid 50s and once again I have discovered it is easy to put weight on. Between my travel, living in Las Vegas (the land of buffets), airport food, and my personal love of cooking, the struggle to revert to old patterns of living resurfaced. The weight I lost after my foot surgery still wanted to come back.

When Victoria sent me an advanced copy of this book to review, I was excited. I was excited because in the six months prior to reading her book, I had finally succeeded in releasing my excess weight and weigh less more healthily than I had over the past decade plus. Now, I feel better, look better, and I have more energy. There is less fear about my health as I age too. I attribute this to my practice of self-hypnosis, in which I use many of the principles Victoria shares in this book. (I also attribute it to Victoria being an amazing accountability partner on the Fitbit app and challenging me to walk more every day!)

This book excites me because it is grounded in a realistic approach to weight loss hypnosis. I shared my story so you can understand how weight loss is not a singular event. For many people, it is a lifelong progression of changes and successes. Far too many hypnotists believe in a magic cure. They promise, "Apply this single technique and voila, you will never be fat again!"

The sessions Victoria outlines in this book are astonishing because they are grounded in what we know works to help people make important changes. It reveals a collection of methods which are research-based, showing lasting and long-term results. I was a bit surprised to see that central to her approach was Progressive Muscle Relaxation (PMR). I was surprised because PMR does not impress other hypnotists at a hypnosis convention, and few hypnotists hold it out in their writings as important. It is often viewed as too slow…too boring…too simple. Yet, research clearly shows that by training clients in the correct way to do PMR profound results are produced.

Those profound results include both emotional, behavioral, and physical changes. Victoria understands the goal of doing hypnotherapy with clients is not to impress other hypnotists at a hypnosis convention with flashy techniques, but rather to produce lifetime results.

The result? She has produced a script book that covers every important topic, from training clients in skill-building hypnosis like PMR, to dealing with emotions and changing lifestyle patterns.

Her ideas, her scripts, her progression through multiple sessions are all testaments to her recognition that equipping clients with skillsets supersedes parlor tricks or hypnotic gimmicks. I believe any hypnotist using this book as a guide and resource will discover how truly life-changing hypnosis for weight loss can be. They will find success with clients that exceeds the promises of pills, potions, processes, and protocols others claim will offer a quick fix.

Best Wishes,

Dr. Richard K. Nongard

Author of *The Seven Most Effective Methods of Self-Hypnosis*
www.SelfHypnosisBook.com
ICBCH Professional Hypnosis www.SubliminalScience.com

Introduction

Who Am I?

Allow me to introduce myself. I'm Victoria M. Gallagher. I'm the founder of a popular hypnosis recording website, called Hyptalk.com. I wrote a book called Practical Law of Attraction which became a #1 best-selling book the day it was released in February of 2019. I'm the founder of HypnoCloud Apps, which is a Hypnosis App giving its users access to over 500 hypnotic recordings. I have written and recorded over 26 comprehensive online courses, hosted at PersonalGrowthClub.com. I became certified in Hypnotherapy in 1999 and that is also when I began my full-time practice.

Prior to becoming a hypnotist, I was a stockbroker. After taking many personal development seminars, I realized my calling was to help people to grow spiritually and work with the power of their mind to create whatever they wanted for themselves. It was always my intention to produce a vast library of personal development resources, and so that is what I set out to do.

Right after opening my office, my branch manager where I worked told me I had 30 days to decide whether to close my business and continue working for the company or quit. I'm thankful I was given that ultimatum. If it wasn't for that, I'm not sure if I would have ever learned how to become a successful entrepreneur.

I mention this only because you may never know exactly what you are capable of achieving with your full potential until you make a decision and are committed to doing so.

If you've been dabbling as a Hypnotherapist and want to go full time, I'm here to tell you, you can do it. You can do anything you set your mind to achieve. My hope is that you will take time to go through this hypnotherapy manual and it will inspire you to create a full-time practice to help people who are desperately in need of changing their lifestyle.

The words I have written in this book, **not only** come from years of wisdom in working with clients, but they also came from years of my own personal struggles with my weight.

I've never been extremely obese. However, I have been a yo-yo dieter my entire life.

Most, no, all of the members of my mom's side of my family have struggled with morbid obesity. I have several relatives who have died as a direct result of obesity related diseases.

When I was around 6 years old, I met one such family member, who eventually died of emphysema and diabetes while still smoking cigarettes and eating massive amounts of sugars and starches. She was an extremely obese 500-pound aunt, my mother's sister.

Seeing this woman, who I knew was related to me, created such a shock to my system. I somehow had this profound awareness. "That could be me when I grow up." I made a decision in that exact moment; I was never going to allow that to happen.

I truly believe in that moment, the shock induced in me a highly hypnotic trance state and that decision I made was a powerful suggestion. Being hypnotized, does not always mean closing your eyes and relaxing. It can take place any time. It is happening all the time. It's happening even by merely living in an environment where you live with people who have accepted their fate to be fat, in pain, poor, addicted, or even depressed. Most of the time, people are living in a trance and unknowingly allowing suggestions to enter their mind which tell them this is just the way it is.

I don't know why I was so lucky to realize this at such a young age. Whatever caused that heightened level of self-awareness, I am grateful and feel truly blessed to have been able to escape the harsh realities I watched most of my mother's side of my family experience.

Even though extreme obesity was never going to be part of my life experience, unfortunately I was not able to get around the tendency to easily gain weight. As such, I deeply empathize with the struggle of trying to keep the weight off. The shame of having a body you're not very proud of. The loss of self-esteem due to beating yourself up over it. The judgement which comes from oneself as well as others who have no tolerance for people who don't look like a Victoria's Secret model. The frustration of not being able to take weight off as easily as it seems it should be. The disappointment of either not reaching the goal in the first place, or reaching that goal only to put back on every bit of weight you lost, plus gain even more.

I also know the feeling of freedom and liberation of being in control of your own healthy choices. I know the feeling of accomplishment of finally reaching your ideal weight and liking the way you look, feel, and the way your clothes fit. Most important, however, is the feeling of self-acceptance and self-love even when you are not in your ideal body. You still have some cellulite, you broke your promise to eat healthy or you missed a day at the gym. You love and accept yourself anyway. You love yourself enough to make a better choice tomorrow.

No one is perfect. There's no such thing as perfection. However, I do believe with a little mental re-conditioning, you can fulfill your potential and create a body you are happy with.

Why is this Program Different?

This program is based on an approach to weight management I successfully applied during one-on-one hypnosis sessions with my clients. I have designed a simple and easy to follow model for using hypnosis to find and resolve core issues responsible for keeping the weight on.

This hypnosis program teaches you how to help your client write their own suggestions they will use which speak to their personal weight loss needs and individual goals.

This program is not only about losing weight, faster and easier than ever before. It is a about creating life-long habits. Becoming physically fit requires the implementation of a number of habits. In this 12-week process, your client will implement a new habit almost every week. Trying to implement all of the habits necessary to maintain weight all at once is only setting oneself up for failure.

In this program, each week, your client will learn a new and easy to implement habit. As your client creates and builds upon these small success's week after week, you are building up your sense of self-confidence as a therapist and so is your client. By the time you complete the program, the material will have become integrated into your client's life for good and you will both feel that success.

As you proceed through each week's session, you are helping your client to gain a deeper understanding of themselves.

Some say it only takes 21 days to create a new habit. Well, experts are now saying it actually takes 90 days to create permanent habits.

The heart of the program is in creating the right affirmations for your client. This is done right from the start during week one. I am going to share my precise formula to create the most effective affirmations for your client.

During the first session or two, you will work together to create these affirmations. You will assign a homework assignment your client will do between sessions. You will implement these affirmations in hypnosis so they will become deeply embedded into their subconscious mind.

While other affirmations in my hypnosis programs are effective, there is no way to create an affirmation which works more powerfully than ones your client will write and say to themselves. These affirmations they write are doubly effective because they are based on their own core limiting beliefs. This is an extremely powerful process, which has been broken down for you in a simple step-by-step process. This will occur over the first week of the program, where we lay down the basic foundation.

Who are You?

You are one of a couple types of people.

You are a Certified Hypnotherapist who works with clients and is looking for ideas and approaches to dealing with weight loss.

As someone in this role, you've been working with clients for quite a while. Maybe you're newer to the field and you're looking for a system. Perhaps you've been in the business for 20 or more years and you're curious to know what methods other accomplished Hypnotherapists have used. It could be that you simply want to organize yourself.

The other reason you are reading this book is because you may have been working in one niche and now you are interested in the world of helping people reach their weight loss goals.

I encourage you to have success in this area. Obesity is a huge and growing epidemic in the country where I live. Over 1/3 of the United States population is now considered obese. There is no shortage of people who deal with this problem. There is, however, clearly a shortage of people who are adept, able, and willing to help resolve the problem.

My hope is that you will become one of those people.

This book does utilize some advanced hypnotherapy techniques. As such, if you are not a clinical Hypnotherapist who's been properly trained by a reputable school, I kindly ask that you do not work with or take money from people until you get the needed training.

If you are an individual who's been through the gamut of trying to lose or maintain weight loss, who still struggles, you too can benefit from this book.

While I initially wrote this book directly for Hypnotherapists, anyone can personally benefit from this book.

You simply follow the same instructions I have given to Hypnotherapists. Instead, direct it toward yourself personally. You can make recordings on your computer or handheld device and listen to them the same way I instruct the Hypnotherapists to tell their clients to do.

If at any point you feel yourself losing the consistency in sticking with the program, I encourage you to seek the help of a properly trained Certified Hypnotherapist, who can guide you through this process. Feel free to share this material with your Hypnotherapist and have them read the book so they can more efficiently and effectively work with you on your journey.

Finally, I reiterate that it's ok to perform self-hypnosis on yourself. It is not ok to use this on other people if you are not trained and certified as a Hypnotherapist.

Setting the Appointment

You want to schedule the first session to be approximately 2 hours and each additional session approximately one hour.

I recommend selling this program to your client as a full package. Many times, clients will either feel they are ready to move on when they are not, or they give up hope if they don't see results right away. Once I started doing programs, and charging them up front, they continued coming to their sessions and they got results.

I believe the one session at a time, especially when it comes to something like weight-loss, is doing your client a disservice. They need a comprehensive plan. They need someone to walk them through a process. They need accountability.

You need to explain to your client on the first session that hypnosis is not magic. It is simply a way to use their mind more effectively and it takes training. It's no different than if they started going to the gym and used a personal trainer who knows how to get specific muscles in shape. You are their personal trainer for their brain. You are their partner helping them achieve their goal.

There will come a time when they will be able to use all the equipment in their mind without you. Maybe it's 10 weeks from now... maybe 12... maybe 24 weeks. In any case, get them to understand that this is a program based on simple successes and how to use their minds and they need to be committed to it. Money is usually the thing that helps people to stay committed to something.

How to Price Your Service

The first thing you need to ask yourself is what is your time worth on an hourly basis.

I still meet Hypnotherapists all the time who undercharge for their time.

As a Hypnotherapist, you are in the business of saving lives, helping people to become healthier, happier, and make better choices in their lives. The people who come to you have usually tried everything else first and failed. Only after seeing a Hypnotherapist, are they able to get rid of things which have caused so much misery, stress, and health problems. You are helping them with what may end up being the most important change they will ever make in their life!

If you're newly starting out and haven't seen many clients yet, sure, you may not feel right to charge much for your services while you are still learning. That's perfectly understandable.

Keep this in mind. People are much more committed to a process they spent a lot of money on than something which didn't cost much.

Perfect example was, the other day I spent $100 to be part of a 5-Day challenge. Something else came up on day 1 of the challenge, which became a much higher priority than the $100 I spent, and I completely blew off the program.

Where money goes priority flows.

The two things to consider when figuring this out is what do you need to make per hour and what is your target audience willing to pay you for your service?

Another way to state this is what is the money motivation factor for them? How much do they need to pay you to be accountable and do the work?

Part of what you charge may depend on where you live. Although these days, you're not limited to seeing clients where you live. You can just as easily set up sessions on Zoom and literally work with people from all over the world.

I'm still seeing rates for sessions, ranging between $75 and $300 per session.

Personally, at this time I charge $250 for an hour and $350 for 90 minutes. People gladly pay this price and feel grateful for my services.

Once you have established what your base hourly price is, then you can begin to create your price for your package.

If you are charging $250 per hour and you offer a 12-week package, you need to offer some sort of incentive for the package. The incentive could be additional things you add to your offer. It could be a discount. Or it could be a combination of both.

I would suggest if you are creating a 12-week or 3-month package, you include a few extras, like access to you by text, email, or a Facebook group. You can add an online course. You can add additional recordings or eBooks. Then, offer anywhere between a 10% - 25% discount for the package.

That would mean considering your 12 hypnosis sessions are valued at $3000 (12 x $250), you could offer it to them for as much as $2700 or as little as $2250.

Will you offer a guarantee?

I will not promise them they will succeed. It is up to them to guarantee their own success. You are a professional and you deserve to be paid for your time. Your value is based on the service you have provided. It's not based on what they choose to do between sessions.

If the program works for even one person, it can work for any person. Yes, lots can be accomplished during the session.

However, to ask to change a lifetime of habits in an hour is ridiculous. They need to have the dedication to reinforce the work you do together during their own time.

How they spend their 6 days or 14 days between the one hour they spend with you makes a huge difference in their level of success. You cannot guarantee how they are going to behave between sessions. It comes down to whether or not they are doing the work you are asking them to do between sessions.

Your time is valuable regardless of what they choose to do after they have come to see you.

Of course, you want them to succeed, so I suggest you work with every resource you have available to help them to get on the path to success.

If you personally have issues with asking people to pay you this kind of money to help them with one of their biggest problems in life, I have a few things for you to consider:

How much do you think they spend on junk food and other ways they are poisoning their bodies?

Do you feel you are worth the money you are asking for?

The helping field seems to have the hardest time asking people to pay them and yet, in my opinion, we help people where it really counts. Think about the other things people spend lots of money on... their cars, computers, clothing, entertainment, traveling, schooling (this is about the best education money can buy!)

Trust me, people have the money to pay you for this valuable service. I rarely have people turn down the opportunity to do work with me for this reason. If they say they don't have the money, it's probably not that important to them and you are not helping them by giving it to them for free. I have done plenty of gratis work and these people that I have worked with for free usually have money allocated toward other things that are more important than their personal growth and well-being.

OK... enough about that. Let's get on with the program.

Beginning with the first contact. When the client contacts you about losing weight, you have a couple of options.

You could simply let them know that you provide a two-hour consultation to see if they are a good fit.

The first consultation is valued at $500, but for a first-time client, I will do it for $250. After meeting with them, I'll have a better understanding of their exact needs and I can suggest a program that best fits them.

This is true because you will know much more about this person at the end of your two-hour session and whether this program is a good fit, or if you need to tailor it more to their unique situation.

The other option is to simply present the program to them during the initial call. However, since they haven't had the experience of hypnosis with you yet, this may require some advanced sales skills, confidence, and that generally comes as a result of working with many clients and having success.

Always take payment at the time you schedule your appointment. Let them know about your 24-hour cancellation policy. They can always call more than 24-hours in advance if they do have an emergency and need to reschedule.

At the end of your first session, since they have already paid the initial payment, you'll present the rest of the program, which you can deduct the initial payment from. You'll say something like: "My packages give you % discount off the price and come with the following added benefits. How would you like to handle that?"

Steer clear from payment plans. Get them to make this commitment to themselves.

In the end, you'll have to play around with what pricing strategy, added benefits, and verbiage works best for you. Whatever you do, do not undervalue yourself or your services. You are not doing anyone any favors by doing this.

Hypnotic Recordings

If you are looking to make recordings for your clients, I strongly recommend you check out my online course called: Passive Profit and Prosperity with Hypnotic Recordings.

To learn more go to: https://www.personalgrowthclub.com/courses/passive-profit-and-prosperity-with-hypnotic-recordings

As a professional hypnosis recording artist since 1999, in that course I cover every single thing you need to know about making hypnosis recordings and selling them on a website for profit, including:

- Choosing Your Niche
- Preparing Your Script
- Recording Studio Setup
- Recording Basics
- How to Use Your Voice Properly
- Backgrounds, Effects, and Binaural Beats
- Editing Techniques
- Product Creation, Pricing, and Packaging
- Graphics
- Product Titles and Descriptions
- Where to Sell Your Recordings
- How to Market Your Website
- Outsourcing

Background Music

Even though you are not selling these recordings you make, you still need to be aware of the copyright laws about recording music. There is plenty of royalty-free music you can buy online for relatively low cost. These are a few places that I have either bought from or that I would buy from in the near future.

https://pond5.com

https://audiojungle.com

https://royaltyfreehypnosismusic.com

https://silenciomusic.co.uk

https://subliminalscience.com/product/royalty-free-music-for-hypnosis-5-hours/

https://highermind-royaltyfreemusic.com/

https://hypnoticmusic.org/

Program Outline

Week 1: The Foundation

During this week, we create the foundation for this program. This week can be broken down into a couple sessions if you want to assist your client with the homework as a second session.

Our objective this week is to:
- Help your client to set a smart goal.
- Teach your client how to go into a hypnotic state using Progressive Muscle Relaxation. (I have included several other induction techniques, such as My Elman, so you can experience different ways of having your client go into trance.)

- Help your client to come up with 10 limiting beliefs, during that session.
- Assign homework, in which they will turn those limiting beliefs into powerful positive affirmations.

Week 2: Hunger Dial

You will help your client learn to detect the difference between real hunger and emotional hunger.

Week 3: Screen of the Mind

In this session your client will work with two screens. A screen with their present weight situation the way it is now and another screen that brings into reality the new behaviors and body they will create.

Week 4: Access the Cause

In this session you will take your client back in time to the root of the problem. Sometimes merely getting an understanding of what's causing weight may help it resolve on its own. This will be a way to find out at an even deeper level, what beliefs are responsible for keeping on this extra weight. At this level of awareness, we invite in new resources to help your client in their endeavors, where they have hindered them in the past.

Week 5: Drinking Water

The effect water has on the body is enormous. The suggestions in this program will help begin weight reduction by drinking water.

Week 6: Exercise

This week we add exercise to the program.

Week 7: Eat Healthy

This week the focus is on healthy eating habits. This is halftime.

Week 8: Metabolism

This week we work with a hypnosis technique to turn up the metabolism and get it working at a level to help to burn calories and increase energy.

Week 9: Banish Old Patterns of Behavior for Good

During this session you will utilize one of the most powerful techniques of Neuro Linguistic Programming. This particular technique was originated by the famous Psychologist, Richard Bandler, and has since been widely used by students of Tony Robbins books and seminars. It's called "Swish." Swishing allows one to switch the representations of things now considered desirable with things that would be more beneficial. Once you learn how to Swish, you can apply this technique to any habit you desire to change.

Week 10: Melt Fat

In this session you will work with the cells within the body.

Week 11: Reshape Your Body

In this session, you work with the outward appearance of the body.

Week 12: Maintenance

This session summarizes everything you have been teaching over the last eleven weeks. These suggestions are about reinforcing the success already achieved, as well as giving additional motivation to keep going.

Assigning Homework

I've briefly mentioned that you will end your sessions by giving your client homework assignments, i.e. listen to the recording, create an affirmation poster, read a hand-out, write in a journal, etc.

Feel free to add to the list of assignments according to your clients' unique needs.

It's important that your client understand the benefits of doing the homework. Establish an agreement with them to do this. Explain the value of them honoring their agreement.

When they break these agreements with you, they are breaking the agreement with themselves. Shed some light on how keeping these agreements to do their homework, will aid in their self-confidence and help them to keep their other agreements in life, such as the decision to exercise or eat healthy.

Listening to the recordings is only going to reinforce the suggestions. You can't break a lifetime of poor habit patterns by listening to something only one time. They need to listen to each weeks' hypnosis recording you are making for them daily.

You'll notice that each week builds upon the last, so I do continue to reinforce the other weeks' information and build it into the current weeks' session.

At the beginning of each session, you'll ask them how the week went. You'll ask them to report any changes in their weight, their hunger, their habits they are working on, and particularly what they agreed to do for themselves that week.

Sometimes your client will come back and haven't done what you've asked them to do.

Week 1: Foundation

(Schedule 2 hours for this first session)

PAPERWORK:

Download Forms and Handouts at www.VictoriaMGallagher.com/wlpbook

During the first hypnosis session, you will need to have ready:

- New file folder for your client.
- Client Agreement form and Policies, which they will sign.
- Smart Goal Sheet.
- Weight Affirmation Handout.
- Create an Affirmation Poster Handout.
- You will keep a notebook and pen handy.

GREETING AND PAPERWORK:

(15 minutes)

Take about 5 minutes to establish rapport with your client. Begin by asking them to tell you a little about themselves. This little chat is important because it gives you an opportunity to mirror them. This is a great NLP technique for getting into relationship with your client and learn their language and style. They may start telling you all about themselves or they may not know what to say at all.

Then, fill out your client agreement. Ask them the questions, and you fill in the information. When you ask them to sign it, ask them to look over the list of policies and sign both sheets.

Next go over the questions in the Weight-Loss Questionnaire. Try to limit the entire paperwork filling time to around 30 minutes.

(I have included samples of these forms. You may use these or re-write them to suit your unique situation.)

After you finish the new client formalities, you are ready to begin the work, starting with setting the foundation.

Step One: Set a Smart Goal

(15 minutes)

Read this over and form your own summary to explain the concept to your client.

Goal setting is one of the most important concepts one can learn. Of course, you have probably at some point set a goal and achieved it before so it's not entirely new to you. However, what we're going to learn about today is a system of goal setting, which will help your client to achieve the goals they set for themselves more often.

Definition of a Goal

I'm going to talk to you briefly about why you want to set a goal in the first place. Then you'll learn an effective way to set a goal. First, let's start with the most basic definition of what a goal is. The definition of a goal is: "The purpose toward which an endeavor is directed." Now why am I defining something as simple as a goal to you when you are thinking that you probably already know what a goal is?

Many people **talk** about setting a goal.

Why do some people achieve their goals and some people don't? I'm going to suggest that it has nothing to do with the actual goal itself or even **how** difficult it would be to achieve it, but rather how the goal is set in the first place.

Going back to our definition; **"The purpose toward which an endeavor is directed,"** as you break this definition down, you may notice there are several key elements to the defined word goal. Let's begin with the first key element; which is **purpose**.

The purpose is simply the desired result. The purpose can be any purpose at all. A purpose can be negative, it can be positive. It can be temporary. It can be permanent. It is simply the result. The more specific the purpose, the more specific the result.

In my practice, I am always asking people what their goals are. What do they want? Here are a few of the more common things I am told. "I want to lose weight." "I want to stop being tired all the time." "I want to get rid of my headaches." Do you hear a common thread among these statements?

The first thing these statements have in common is that they are all stated in the negative. The next thing that they have in common is that they all are talking about something that they don't want. What am I saying by stated in the negative? I'm saying that there are negative words involved in these sentences. **Lose** is a negative word. **Stop** is a negative word. **Get Rid** is a negative phrase. Finally, they are not specific.

Now, do I mean you should never use these words or that they are bad words? No! What I do mean is that if you have negative words in your goal or in your affirmations or in your self-talk, it is likely that you are drumming up a picture or idea or concept in your mind of "weight", "headache", or "tired" as in these examples.

Since your subconscious mind cannot differentiate between a negative phrase or a positive phrase, it's only going to bring you more of whatever that thought is. You see the weight in your mind when you say lose weight. You see tired all the time when you think tired. You think about headaches when you think the word headache.

"Pink Bunny"

Give your client the example of trying not to think about something, such as a pink bunny or a yellow lemon. Keep repeating it to them; "don't think about the pink bunny. Whatever you do, do not think about the pink bunny." Then ask them what picture they had in their mind. They will likely tell you they were thinking about a pink bunny.

Be Specific

Goals can be phrased in a positive way and still not yield the results you want. For example: "I want to have more money." Since I am so generous, this is one we don't even need hypnosis for. I reach into my purse; I grab my wallet and I give them exactly what they have asked for: more money. I hand them one shiny penny and I say, your wish is my command, and you now have more money. Is there anything else you want? Some say, "I want to feel better." I ask what is better? What does better feel like? And why would you want to feel it?

Don't let your client get away with this! You are wasting your time and your client's time if you let them tell you that they want more or better. You've got to get specific with them. You will notice this is not an easy thing to do. The more you give your clients these analogies and explain to them that your subconscious mind has no idea what these words mean to them, they will start to get it and give you the specific information. This goal setting technique will be an ideal way to help you get it too.

Money Analogy

Most people will simply say, "Well, you know what I mean." And the honest truth is that, you don't know what they mean. One can only guess or assume what they mean. Using the money analogy again, more money could mean $100 a month more or it could mean $1,000,000 in your bank account. It could mean $1 billion a year more. Sometimes people know, themselves, how much more they mean, but for some reason they won't say it. Maybe because they feel embarrassed or foolish to ask for what they really want.

For most people however, they have never sat down and figured out precisely what they want. If they don't know what they want, you certainly don't know either. By always asking them to be more specific, you are helping them to discover more about themselves. Remind them that their subconscious mind does the best to produce the result that best matches what they have been directing it to think about.

They say you are exactly where you want to be in life, and I hold a belief that this is mostly correct. I believe that deep down, people probably want something different than what they have now. They just didn't know how to talk to their brains in such a way that it will help them produce the results they want.

Sports Analogy

Here's another way to think about a goal. In sports or games, there is a clear forward-thinking purpose and an endeavor. Cross the finish line. Score the most points. Or knock out your opponent. Do you ever hear them say, my goal is to not lose? Or score more? Get rid of my obstacles?

Ask your client specifically, "What is your goal? What specific result are you aiming toward?" Their purpose can be anything. It can be simply to complete the program. It can be to weigh a specific amount by the end of the program. It can be to make healthy a present health issue; creating a healthy blood sugar level of…. Or reducing their blood pressure to a healthy level of … Other specific goals regarding health and weight could be body fat percentage. It could be measurements. It could be the size of clothes they are wearing. It could be the amount of times per week they will work out or walk. It could be the amount of times per day they drink water. It could be the % of time they eat healthy food.

Once you get their initial goal, write it down and you will be testing it against the S.M.A.R.T. goal setting system.

You will also get an agreement from them that they will get an accurate starting point of where they are presently.

Now, let's look at another element to a goal. Endeavor. The endeavor part of the goal is simply that thing that one is doing about their purpose. It's whatever conscious effort or action they will be taking.

This program provides one of the ways to endeavor toward that purpose.

A goal is a purpose, an endeavor, and finally it is directed. The endeavor has got to be something that moves them in the direction toward the purpose of their goal.

Why should you set a goal?

First, there are already unconscious goals in place that they probably aren't aware of. Let's say their desire is to be 25 pounds thinner. In other words, they currently weigh 25 pounds more than they would like. If they are 25 pounds overweight, that has been their unconscious goal up until now. This is unconscious. What setting a goal does is it provides an opportunity to consciously direct endeavors toward a new purpose.

Let's discuss how to go about setting a goal. How you will know that your clients' goal is a goal, is that it will meet the criteria I will now outline.

Here are the 5 criteria the goal will meet: It's easy to remember the 5 criteria because the acronym spells out the word smart.

"**S**" stands for specific. I've already given you a lot of information so far about specific. However, one other thing I'll mention about specific is that they should be able state it clearly in one or two sentences. Remember to have them state their goal in the positive, what they *want*, not what they don't want. Another thing I suggest is beginning the goal with the words "I am." "I am" is the most powerful sentence in the English language.

"**M**" stands for Measurable, does the goal give a specific way to measure it. Specific and measurable can be stated in the same words. For example, if the goal is to weigh 125 pounds, that is specific, and it is measurable. You have to have a way to access whether the desired results have been achieved or not.

"**A**" stands for Achievable. Does the client believe they can do it? Is this a realistic goal? This is tricky and should be balanced with the "R" part of the acronym, which is realistic. You want to have your client set a goal that they will achieve, even if it's something you have never done before or don't know yet how you will achieve it.

"**R**" stands for Realistic. Can the goal be reached within the given timetable? Does the client have the commitment needed in order to reach their goal? Is there excitement and something to keep them motivated toward achieving new heights in their life? On the other hand, if their goal is only 5 pounds, that's probably a little too realistic and not too exciting. On the other hand of its 100 pounds in 12 weeks, we need to access whether they are setting themselves up for failure.

"**T**" stands for Timetable. Goals need to fall within a certain time frame, otherwise they are never achieved, and likely never to even get started. Putting the goal into a time frame will help them to stay on track toward achieving their goals. For the purpose of THIS goal that they will be setting, I suggest you use a 12-week time frame. While they may have a longer-term goal, I suggest chunking it down into smaller goals achieved in smaller timetables.

Remember, the goal you will help them write will be in one or two sentences. Write on your paper S M A R and T and make sure that you can answer yes and put a little check mark next to each of those letters before moving on to the next step.

When you have completed writing down your goal ask your client to sign the document and to specifically say their goal out loud to 5 people between now and their next session. This will be a great way for them to reinforce their goal from the very beginning. They have not only made an agreement with you, but they have also made it with themselves and with those people, who will likely want to support them.

Step Two: Progressive Muscle Relaxation and Negative Beliefs

Next, you will teach your client how to go into a hypnotic state, using progressive muscle relaxation and working at a subconscious level you will assist your client in getting the negative core thought patterns to surface. During the hypnosis session and when they come out, you will write down the negative beliefs they tell you.

After you get all ten of these negative beliefs, you will be helping them to convert these negative beliefs into positive affirmations.

You will be working with these positive affirmations during this and later hypnosis sessions. I'll be talking more about these negative beliefs and positive affirmations momentarily.

Pre-Talk

(15 minutes)

Here is a good pre-talk you can use before beginning the hypnosis session:

What we're going to do in the next few moments is the most elementary basic technique for teaching your body how to become relaxed. It's called progressive muscle relaxation. The reason we are going to use this particular technique is because I know that it is a bona fide surefire way for you to experience relaxation taking place in your body. There are many other techniques for getting you into a hypnotic state just as well, if not even better, but for these first couple of sessions, let's **give** your body 100% of your attention.

What is Progressive Muscle Relaxation?

It is simply a tensing and relaxing of your muscles in progression from either top to bottom or from bottom to top. You will physically tense each muscle we come to, hold the muscle tight for about 5 seconds, then release the muscle.

The reason this process is guaranteed to work is because of a basic physiological principal. When you create tension in a muscle and then release that tension, the muscle has no choice but to relax. In other words, the muscle is not going to stay locked in that tense state that you intentionally put it into, no, it's going to relax.

One interesting aspect about this process is that this muscle relaxation goes a step further and it will not only go back to the level of relaxation it was before you tensed it, it will become even more relaxed than before. As we apply the tensing and releasing technique to each of your muscles, you will notice other changes naturally occur in your body. For example, you become calm. Your breathing slows down. Your heart rate slows down. Most importantly, when you relax this way your mind becomes open and receptive to suggestions.

A couple of words about hypnosis and then we'll go ahead and get started. Many times, people report that they don't feel like they were hypnotized. I ask, if you were hypnotized, how would it have felt?

If this is your first time with hypnosis, then here is what I ask. Do not expect to feel any different than you do right now. Just a little more relaxed. Hypnosis can be an elusive feeling. When you experience it at first, sometimes you are not aware that what you are experiencing is actually hypnosis.

You may not feel extremely deep levels when you are first getting started. However, the truth is, most changes do not require a deep level of hypnosis. Most of what we are going to work with will deal with your ability to concentrate. Instead of worrying about whether you think you are hypnotized or not, just think about deeply concentrating on what I am saying to you.

WEEK 1

Please don't put any expectations on yourself to feel any of the ways you might think hypnosis is supposed to feel. If you haven't experienced it before it's likely not going to feel like you think it will.

On the other hand, after a period of time, you will come to know a certain familiarity that goes along with whatever state you do experience. You will realize there's a certain subtle feeling you get that tells you when you are in it.

Sometimes people get a little too drowsy in hypnosis and they fall asleep and they ask if this is still effective. I say it is still having some impact on your subconscious mind, in much the same way that television has some impact on your mind if you fall asleep to it.

However, while the subconscious mind is 90% of your mind AND is the more powerful part of your mind, you need your conscious mind alert, awake, and focused in order to assimilate the suggestions I give you and to draw the pictures I ask you to draw. Do whatever you need to do to keep yourself awake.

I am going to ask you to come up with a list of your 10 negative suggestions that keep you in your negative behaviors.

Let me explain what I am looking for. Please use your own thoughts when developing these. What I am looking for are those reasons you give yourself that keep you doing what you want to stop doing. For example, let's say junk food is your problem and you pass by the junk food place and decide to get some against your better judgment. What is that thing that you say to yourself that makes it ok for you to do it?

These are the beliefs that are **in favor of your unhealthy habits**. For example, **"I just don't have time to eat right."** Or **"I'll just do it one more time and then I'll do better tomorrow."** Or **"This food is not that bad."** Please come up with your own list of ten and I am going to have you go into hypnosis to get in touch with those moments so you can hear those thoughts happening as they happen for you.

Usually at about 4 or 5 items on the list, a client will say, "there just aren't any more." I tell you this, **there are *more* than 10** benefits for your unhealthy behaviors, otherwise you wouldn't be doing it. Trust me on this.

Remember, as you are making this list of 10 things, these are the thoughts that **support your poor eating or exercise habits. "I don't feel like working out." "I don't like the gym." "I don't have the time."** Whatever is true for you. We need to get in touch with those limiting beliefs so we can address them.

Everyone I have ever worked with had a hard time making this list at first, and everyone I have ever worked with was able to come up with all ten by the end of their first session with me.

Why is this hard? **These thoughts are unconscious!!** You don't usually hear yourself making these justifications to yourself. You do it usually unconsciously. This is one of the greatest steps toward change is to **become aware of what some of those thoughts are.**

Important! Note to Hypnotherapist:

This script serves two purposes.

1. When you are with your client on their first session, it is used for the purpose of gathering their negative beliefs.

    You do not want to record the questions or answers you are asking your client so you will stop the recording and start the recording again when you are given instructions to start.

2. This is the recording your client will continue listening to after their first session with you. They will use this recording for the purpose of giving themselves the positive suggestions you will help them create after they awaken from trance.

Say to your client before you put them into trance:

"I'm going to ask you to open your eyes and read your positive suggestions. Today, you will tune out that command as it only applies to the work you'll be doing on your own after today's session. I will let you know when it's time to tune in to me again. Does that make sense?"

WEEK 1

Once you have told the client what to expect, it is now time to begin recording.

Make note of the place for you to stop recording and the place for you to start again.

Progressive Muscle Relaxation

(30 minutes)

In a moment ... you'll be relaxing every muscle in your body... which will cause you to feel a beautiful sense of calm and peace ... in your body ... your mind ... your emotions ... and your soul ... a wonderful feeling that you'll be able to bring forth whenever you think about it ... from this point forward.

Many people spend their whole lives in search of this kind of peace of mind ... you'll be creating for yourself in the next little while ... Even though you may have never experienced such a depth of relaxation as you are about to experience ... Give yourself this time ... to experience yourself ... to experience lightness ... weightlessness ... pleasure. It's so important that you take time to do this...

Each day you allow yourself this opportunity ... to go within ... you will achieve deeper states than ever before ... and you will be able to access a state of trance more quickly and easily.

Let's begin.

By now, you will have adjusted your body into a comfortable quiet place where you will remain undisturbed for the next 25 minutes. You can sit in a chair with your back straight and your feet firmly planted in front of you or lie down, whichever works better for you and is more comfortable ... so long as you will remain slightly awake throughout this entire process ... Keep your arms and legs uncrossed in an open body position.

Tune into your breathing ... place one hand on your lower abdomen ... when you breathe, make sure that your breath is filling up your entire abdomen and that you are breathing slowly ... Inhaling to a slow count of four ... then holding that breath ... and exhaling to a slow count of eight

Take a moment to pay attention to your breathing ... and imagine that you are breathing in relaxation and breathing out any tension or stress ... I'll be silent for one minute to give you some time to practice breathing in such a way that your abdomen is rising and falling with each breath.

(Pause one minute)

Breathe naturally. Notice your level of relaxation, which is getting deeper and deeper all the time.

Direct your attention to the top of your head... to your scalp ... to the skin that covers your scalp ... feel this area and notice any of the sensations in this area around the top of your head.

You may notice your pulsation at the top of your head, or you may notice a tingling sensation. Do whatever you need to do to cause this part of your body, the top of your head to become calm and relaxed. Focus on your forehead. Cause your forehead to become tense by raising your eyebrows and hold that position for the next 5 seconds... and now relax your forehead... feel your forehead smoothing out and becoming limp and relaxed.

Place your attention on your eyes and close your eyes tightly. Hold for a count of 5. Relax your eyes. Let go of all the tiny little muscles that surround your eyes. Allow this part of your body to relax deeper.

Direct all your attention now to your jaw muscles. Cause this part of your body to become tense by clinching your teeth together, holding for a few seconds... and relax your jaw completely... you allow your jaw to become even more relaxed by allowing your lips and your teeth to part slightly. Allow your jaw go limp and droop down and relax.

This is a wonderful signal to help the rest of your body relax as well. Moving down your body, let yourself feel any tension in the back of your neck by slowly bending your neck back and hold that tension for 5 seconds. Release the tension in your neck by taking in a deep breath, let your neck fall naturally into a comfortable position and expel all the air from your lungs.

Breathe out any remaining feelings of tightness. Relax your neck.

Now we come to the shoulders, another area where you might store a lot of your tension. Feel that tension by bringing your shoulders upward toward your ears and hold. Breathe in again and let your shoulders drop down to a position that feels perfect. As you breathe out, become even more relaxed as your shoulders rest comfortably in their relaxed position. When your body relaxes this way; your mind and your emotions follow along and become just as relaxed while you focus all of your attention on relaxing each of these muscles in your body.

You will now focus your attention on your arms. Feel the muscles in your upper arms and your lower arms. Tense these muscles by stretching your arms downward, alongside your legs, stiffening and tensing the muscles within your arms and hold. Release your arms. Let them go loose and limp. Imagine all the energy drain out of your arms, so you feel that you couldn't lift them even if you tried.

We now come to your hands. Cause your hands to become tense by making a fist. Hold that fist tight for a moment... Release the tension. Feel the warmth and relaxation spreading throughout your hands and your fingers. You might even feel a slight tingling sensation.

Turn your attention toward the muscles in your back area. Cause these muscles in your back to become tense by pushing your shoulders back a little and feel that tension for about 5 seconds. Release it. Let go of your back and let relaxation run throughout that entire area. Focus on your chest by taking in and holding a deep breath. Breathe in and hold your breath to a count of five and when you let the breath out, let your lungs and your chest feel the relief of relaxation.

Just breathe naturally and let each breath that you take from now on cause you to drift into a deeper state of relaxation. What a beautiful, healthy state of calm, which is becoming deeper all the time.

Now, focus on your abdomen and squeeze the muscles of your abdomen, suck in those muscles, feel them tight and tense...

hold... and release them. Feel them more and more relaxed. Feel your breath sending waves of relaxation into your belly. Feel it and go even deeper. Next, tense the muscles of your buttocks. Squeeze your buttocks muscles and hold. Let them go. Relax your buttocks muscles.

Direct your focused attention to your thighs. Tighten these muscles in your thighs for a few seconds. Release your thighs completely. Let them go completely loose and limp. Feeling good, feeling relaxed and now your calves... tense these muscles in your calves and hold the tension... and release the tension.

Feel the waves of comfort and relaxation which have spread throughout your entire body and you will now go into an even deeper state of relaxation by paying close attention to your feet. Feel your feet and point your toes as if you were squeezing out that last little bit of tension ... hold it for a moment... as you let your feet go and let them relax completely.

Imagine yourself as an energy. That can look like anything you like. This energy that has been inside of this body and that you could just float up, right out of your body. Allow your body to let go and rest peacefully, while you, the real you, the purest essential part of your being, which you may call your spirit, or whatever feels best for you, this part of you will float and let your body be. Just float up and leave your body so it can receive the most benefit from this relaxation. Your mind and your emotions are leaving your body, so your body can rejuvenate itself.

Imagine yourself in any way you wish, that you are just energy, your spiritual self, looking down at your body which is sitting or lying so peacefully. You're up there above your body about six feet or so. You now draw a brilliant illuminating white protective light all around your body. You may want to add some color to this white light like purple flecks or gold sparkle. While you see yourself with this glowing beautiful light all around you, you feel much more peaceful and relaxed.

You will remain in this dreamy drowsy state for as long as you like or until the time when I ask you to bring your attention back to waking consciousness. At the time I ask you to come back to full waking consciousness, you will become aware of your body again and everything will return back to normal. For now, you'll simply continue to let everything in this physical realm go completely.

My voice brings you deeper and deeper into relaxation. Allow my voice to affect and become your own internal voice. The words I say to you from now on will have a profound effect on you. My words will strongly influence your thoughts, your behaviors, your feelings, and help you to make the changes in your life that you desire to make. The more you listen, the more influence my voice will have upon you and the deeper you will go into hypnosis.

Your subconscious mind hears my words and these words become your predominant thoughts. All of your old thoughts, which promote negative behaviors, lose any of the power you once gave them. You may hear a negative thought, and you are now able to turn down the volume on that thought and turn up the volume on the thoughts that support you in creating what you desire. This state of relaxation is the most powerful state you can experience.

You were born with the most amazing tool ever known to man, your subconscious mind, where you can create anything you want. It's always nice to have someone guide you into this state, but please know that you have created this simply by listening and following the instructions. You can always come here to this place of relaxation any time you want. Use this tool for yourself. Use it often. It is your gift. It is within you.

You are an amazing human being. You are powerful. You can and you will achieve whatever you desire. Let's now have a moment of silence so that you can go within yourself and experience yourself more completely.

(Pause one minute, then continue with the Negative Belief Script.)

Download your scripts at www.VictoriaMGallagher.com/wlpbook

Negative Beliefs Script

Your mind is powerful and is capable of doing many wonderful things. Over the next few days, weeks, and months you are going to be learning new things, mainly how to use your subconscious mind to make permanent changes in your body. Your subconscious mind stores all of your emotions, behavior patterns, habits, and memories. It only knows how to do what it has been programmed to do. It tends to perform only the commands that have a strong influence on it. The only way your subconscious mind can now become strongly influenced is through repetition or emotion.

As you listen to this program, experience it as best as you can and listen to it many times, so we are taking care of both repetition and emotion.

READ Affirmations to p.36

(Stop the recording here and continue on with the rest of the script.)

Some time ago you have had other ideas, which have influenced your subconscious thinking today. This thinking is the part of you, which has insisted on you giving in to your cravings and your binges. It's the part of you, which has lied to you in some way, and told you it would be all right to snack on this or have just one more, or whatever those words are for you.

While you are in this state and relaxing deeper and deeper, you're going to call upon those things that you have told yourself. Those negative suggestions that you have given to yourself or that you have given in to. Reach deep inside and find those limiting beliefs that have been causing you to gain weight. I'll be giving you some time to think about this.

One way that may make it easy for you to get in touch with these negative beliefs is to ask yourself the who, what, when, where, why, and how questions: For example, when do I eat? And if you hear yourself saying, I eat when I am bored, or I eat when I am upset, that might be one of your negative triggers.

Another example might be "Why do I eat?" Here you may hear something like, "I eat to reward myself," or "I eat to give myself love." At this time. Go inside. Go deeper inside your mind. Experience yourself during some of those times when you have eaten the foods you didn't need to eat or when you have eaten too much or too fast, or whatever it has been for you. As you imagine those times, get in touch with those experiences.

I'm going to ask you some questions. You'll be able to speak and answer my questions out loud, while remaining in hypnosis.

- *How are you physically feeling while you are overeating?*
- *As you are seeing yourself and experiencing yourself there, put some emotion in that scene.*
- *What are the emotions you experience while you are eating?*
- *What emotions are being disguised?*
- *What emotions were you feeling before you started eating? (It doesn't have to be negative emotions. Some people eat when they feel happy or excited.)*
- *What are the words that you could put with those feelings and images?*
- *What are some things you might be saying to yourself?*
- *What are the permissive words which make it ok for you to eat in this way?*
- *What kind of excuses are you making?*
- *Make sure you are honest with yourself. The more you get to the heart of these negative suggestions you have been giving yourself the easier it will be to create the correct suggestions that are going to help you to succeed at your weight goal.*
- *I am going to be giving you a few moments to allow those beliefs to come into your awareness now. If you have any other thoughts like this come to you while in this state, please feel free just to shout them out at any moment.*

(Pause one minute)

Good, in a moment, I'm going to ask you to open your eyes on the count of three.

Like we talked about before, just tune that out this time around and rest peacefully for a few moments, until you hear me say the following words:

"Rest into a deep hypnotic state."

When you hear me say, "Rest into a deep hypnotic state," that is your queue to tune into my suggestions again.

Nod your head if you understand.

(Begin recording again here.)

Now when I count to 3, while remaining in a hypnotic state, open your eyes and read your new positive suggestions. I will give you a few moments of silence to allow you to let the suggestions sink in. When you have all ten of your suggestions memorized and feel like you would rather do this with your eyes closed that would be fine too. You simply bypass the suggestions for opening your eyes.

Now on the count of three, you will open your eyes. You will feel slightly out of it and groggy, but you will be aware enough to receive and accept the suggestions you have written down for yourself. 1. 2. 3. Open your eyes and read your suggestions.

(If they open their eyes while in this first session, simply have them close their eyes and relax for a few moments and try not to get that recorded.)

(Pause two minutes – long enough for them to read each of their ten positive affirmations.)

(Proceed normally.)

Good, now you can set your affirmations aside and let go and rest back into a deep hypnotic state. Good and go deeper. Every time you hear me mention the word deeper you will feel yourself resting even deeper than before. Go deeper. Good. Resting ever so deeply. Deeper. You are changing your life for good and permanently. Your new suggestions are implanting themselves in every cell of your body and creating the wonderful positive benefits you want them to create.

Whenever you are tempted to engage in your old core negative thinking, you will immediately hear these new suggestions you have created for yourself. These new positive suggestions become your new way of thinking. You accept these suggestions quickly and easily. These new changes are taking affect and become your present reality. You are powerful. You have a positive attitude. You are feeling better about yourself every day in every way.

(Trance termination)

Download your scripts at www.VictoriaMGallagher.com/wlpbook

Trance termination

Now if it's time for sleep, allow yourself to drift off into dreamy drowsy deep sleep and you will simply bypass any of the remaining suggestions for waking. If it is time for you to come back to full waking consciousness, you will do so at the count of 5, feeling relaxed and well rested, like you are waking up from a nice long nap. If you are ready to come back, you'll come up slowly and gently at the count of 5.

Number one. You are beginning to feel your body where it has been resting so still and quiet and notice the blood flow begin to pick up its pace a little, perhaps by noticing a tingling in your fingers, your head or your toes. Number two. Waking up even more. Good ... feel your body emerging from its restful state into a wakeful energetic state. Good ... and three. That's right you are ready to be wakeful, so breathe in the wakeful energy and breathe out any feelings of being tired. Notice how good it feels to become wakeful again. Number four, almost there.

Move your arms and your legs, wiggle your fingers and toes and stre-e-e-tch out your torso. Good. Now five. Eyes wide open. You are fully alert and ready to be responsive and energetic. You have all your energy and you are perfectly wide awake.

Give the client a little time to get coherent again and assess their experience.

(Take notes)

If you have not written 10 negative beliefs down at this point, you will need to work with your client further to finish the list. Ask your client if there were more negative thoughts that came to them during that last part of the session. Continue prompting them for more until you have the list created.

Step Three: Create Powerful Positive Affirmations:

You will teach your client to create their own personal set of powerful positive affirmations.

Now, you are going to help your client take those negative beliefs and turn them into powerful positive affirmations. Why are they powerful? They are directly speaking to the core issue.

There are a number of rules in creating these affirmations. Discuss this with your client so they understand. Have them make the affirmations. You can help them along, but make sure they own them. This is the foundation of the program is that they have created the affirmations themselves. Empower them. Yes! They are capable of doing this no matter how confused they say they are about it.

You have your notepad with their negative beliefs. You read one off at a time.

They have a notepad and they will write their own list in their own handwriting of the positive counter to that negative belief.

How to Convert Negative Beliefs into Positive Powerful Affirmations?

We're going to take this list of 10 negative beliefs and turn them into positive powerful affirmations. You are going to make this list. Let's imagine that you have a positive self and a negative self. Your negative self wants to keep you in your old behavior. As such, it will likely put up a little fight to keep you doing those things. What you will do is for each of these 10 statements we just made, imagine this is your positive self, speaking up for you and what you would like now. There are a few things we have to keep in mind when creating these new affirmations.

1. You must remember to talk about what you want to add to your life here, not what you want to take away.
2. Affirmations must be stated in the positive. Let me give you an example. Here was your negative belief: "I always have to stop for fast food on my way home." Let's start with an incorrect example. An ineffective positive affirmation would be, "I never stop for fast food anymore." What's wrong with this affirmation? (Wait for their answer.)

   The idea of this affirmation is fast food. You still get a picture of the fast food, right? Whatever you think about, you will attract. What do you want to attract? A healthy habit.

   Keep in mind that nature abhors a vacuum, if you take away a bad habit, i.e. stopping for fast food, that void will be replaced, however you can choose to replace it with whatever you want instead of letting nature fill it at random. The idea was to replace this negative belief with a positive affirmation.
3. Next, phrase affirmations in the present tense. Take out the word "will" or "am going to" from your vocabulary. Even "want." What these words leave you with is exactly what you are stating, a want or that it will happen sometime in the future. This will never happen since it is sometime in the future.
4. Finally, the affirmation must be believable. You may not do it or have it at this moment, but is it something you can believe?

Following these four rules here is our old negative belief:

"I always have to stop for fast food on my way home."

And here are some examples of how this negative belief can be converted to a powerful positive affirmation:

FOUNDATION

"I now prefer to stop for healthy foods."

"I like the way stopping for healthy foods makes me feel."

"Stopping for healthy foods is a satisfying choice."

Do you get the idea? Have your client say the affirmation they are going to write down so you can make sure that all 10 of you're the positive affirmations follow the rules. Sometimes, you can let things slide. However, there are certain words to make absolutely sure you don't have in your affirmations.

First and foremost, you don't want to include the idea of whatever it is you are wanting to eliminate, i.e. the laziness, the bad foods. Change those ideas to the positive ideas you want to have. This can be challenging sometimes, only because we are so in the habit of focusing on what we don't want, that we have forgotten how to think about what we do want.

Here's a list of words to avoid in these statements. I could go into a whole recording about why to avoid these words. For now, trust me on this:

- Not
- Don't
- Try
- Can't
- But
- Hope
- Attempt
- Failure
- Better
- Bad
- Right
- Wrong
- Should
- Shouldn't
- Worse
- Hurt
- Pain
- Wont

VICTORIA M. GALLAGHER

In a nutshell, these words either invite the negative thing into your sentence. Or they make a judgment about something, that will likely result in self-judgment.

By the end of today's session, your client now has their ten new positive affirmations and you will assign the following homework.

HOMEWORK:

- State S.M.A.R.T. goal to five people.
- Listen to recording every day
- Create an Affirmation poster (bring it to next session)
- Get a three-ring binder and do all assigned homework in a journal, bring to each session. Keep all handouts in the three-ring binder. (You could provide them a 3-ring binder with some kind of design with your logo on the front of it.)

Create an Affirmation Poster

What you'll need for homework are the following supplies: your notebook and pen, some inspiring music you like, colored pens or crayons, a piece of 8 1/2 by 11 or 11 by 14 white or light colored poster board, glue, a fitness magazine or two, and a pair of scissors.

After you have your list together, you'll then beautifully and creatively write them on your poster board with the colored pens and crayons. Cut a few images or words from your fitness magazine and paste them around your poster board. Get it just the way you like it.

Keep this poster board in the same location that you'll be doing your hypnosis every day. Someplace where you have easy access to it, and you can see it easily. Before beginning and after each day's hypnosis session, spend one minute looking at your poster board, the pictures, and the affirmations. If you feel drawn to do so, you may add new images or quotes or your own new affirmations to it along the way. You may feel like you need to change an affirmation, so it applies to you more. You may find an affirmation on one of the programs that you'll hear that you like and want to add it to your board. Just in case, when you make this board, be sure to leave room so you can add to it later.

Homework is an important part of the program. Do not underestimate the power of this simple tool. It works. Sometimes it's the simplest things in life that have the most power.

Week 2: Hunger Scale

PAPERWORK:

Download Handouts at www.VictoriaMGallagher.com/wlpbook

During the second hypnosis session, you will need to have ready:

- Hunger Scale Diagram.
- Emotional Eating Journal.

FOLLOW-UP FROM LAST WEEK:

- Ask client to see the affirmation poster they made.
- Ask client what their smart goal is and if they told 5 people about it.
- Ask client how many times they listened to their recording.
- Make sure they brought their journal.

Education about the Hunger Scale

HANDOUT:

- Hunger Scale Diagram

This week we are going to introduce a new tool that you'll be using throughout this program called: The Hunger Scale. A hunger scale is simply an intuitive way to prevent you from overeating. The hunger scale teaches you how to listen to your body. The goal is to become mindful of your eating. That is to be more in control of your eating by listening to your bodies' natural signals for food and to stop eating when your body is full.

We eat for many reasons other than hunger. It can be due to boredom, stress, habit, being tired, thirst, or as a reward. Yes, believe it or not, thirst can be confused with hunger.

One of the best things you can do for your body is to drink water, which we're going to be getting into more of later in this program. If you are not sure about your hunger, I suggest drinking a refreshing glass of water first and then see how you feel.

Being tired or run down can also make you think you are hungry. Make sure you are getting adequate rest.

Stress can be reduced significantly simply by going into a state of hypnosis on a daily basis.

Of course, there are plenty of healthy ways you can reward yourself. You can treat yourself to a new recording or a hot bubble bath. You can also create positive habits for yourself when you feel like eating, like going for a 15-minute walk, calling a friend, or writing in a journal.

In this hypnosis session, you are going to learn how to work with your body so that it will tell you when you are truly hungry and when you are not. In your notebook this week, you'll jot down those times when you were not really hungry. Make a note of what it is that you are feeling and what you actually wanted. This is a wonderful way to acknowledge any unmet needs you may have and that will help you to break the cycle of eating when you're not hungry.

Hunger Scale Script

(Induction)

It's likely, at times in your past, you have eaten when you weren't physically hungry. Instead, you were psychologically hungry, meaning, you have learned a response to certain emotions, and by habit, you have fulfilled whatever was unconsciously missing with food.

The classic case of this is eating out of boredom. How many times have you gone to the refrigerator, standing there with the door wide open, wondering what you should eat? You weren't really hungry. You were simply bored. It may have become a habit to eat when you felt bored or during other times when you weren't hungry.

You desire to become healthy. Not only physically healthy, but also emotionally and mentally healthy as well. You now desire to replace these old habits with these new positive healthy habits that I will be sharing with you in the next few moments. We're going to teach your subconscious mind how to let you know when your hunger is real or if there's some other need it is trying to satisfy.

Let's take a little tour inside your brain. Imagine the inside of your head. Notice how way deep inside; there is a control room. As your curiosity begins to take over, you begin moving closer to the control room inside your mind, and you notice a room filled with the most magnificent technology you have ever seen. You are amazed to notice things you never even thought about before. There are temperature gauges that cause your body to heat up or cool down. There's a dial that controls the speed of your heartbeat. There's even a little switch that turns on and controls your sweat glands.

You are amazed when you realize all the things that go on in this little secret room in your mind you never even realized existed before. Nor were you ever aware you had access to such a place in your mind. After you have taken a good look around at all the cool things you now know you can come back and work on any time you need to, you'll then locate a particular area in your control room called your hunger scale. This is a scale that gauges your actual physical hunger that you feel in your body and it is numbered 1 through 10. Find it yet?

On your hunger scale, notice the number 1 position is starving, and the number 10 position is stuffed. Bring to mind a time when you felt you were at a number 1, starving; get in touch with how that feels. Good. Recall a time when you felt you were at a number 10, stuffed. Notice how that feels. Good.

Now that you have experienced both ends of the spectrum, let that be the last time you ever feel starving or stuffed. There is a point between 1 and 10 when you will begin to eat.

Now move to a 3 on your hunger scale and notice that feeling. Any time you feel yourself at a 3, you begin to eat. From now on, you eat slowly, and you now become aware of your body's physical need for food the entire time while eating. You are a little bit surprised to notice that you receive more enjoyment and fulfillment during this controlled time of eating.

Now move to a 7 on your hunger scale and notice the way 7 feels. Here you are completely satisfied and content to stop eating.

Imagine yourself at a point in time when you are hungry. During this week, you now create the habit of detecting your hunger level. Whenever you think about eating from this point forward, ask yourself this simple question, "How hungry am I?" This question, immediately calls up the hunger scale within your control room and you either see an answer, feel an answer, or hear an answer from within. It only takes a few seconds.

Once again, you now create a habit that at any point you ever think about eating or find yourself getting ready to eat or sense hunger, immediately before making any movement toward food of any sort, you ask the simple question, "how hungry am I?" and your body gives you the answer. From now on, you will eat only if you are at or below a 3 on your hunger scale. From this point on, you eat slowly, savoring and enjoying every morsel of food, and you stop eating at a 7. You simply want to stop there. Your body is learning now to give you a clear hunger signal at a 3. Your body from this point forward, persistently alerts you of your hunger as soon as you get to a 3.

You are learning to become more sensitive to listening to your body and you desire to work with your body so that it works optimally for you. You are happy to get a clear signal to slow down and to stop eating when you're full. If you are ever eating at a pace which makes it difficult for you to detect whether your body is becoming satisfied or not, you will hear a clear and direct signal coming from inside of you to slow down. I'll give you a moment to imagine this happening. This signal may come to you in the form of a yellow light or you may suddenly become sensitive to the way your belly feels, or you may hear the words, slow down.

Take a moment to imagine how that is going to happen for you.

(Pause 30 seconds)

Good. From now on, whenever you get the feeling of a 7, you will stop eating. You will know that this scale is accurate when you find yourself eating about 5 times a day, small portions of food. This is the way your body likes to be fed. You want to be kind to your body by feeding it the way it wants to be fed.

This week you are in the habit of detecting your hunger level, by asking the question, "How hungry am I?" hearing the answer within and responding to your body's natural request for food when your hunger scale is at a 3.

Let's imagine another time when you are thinking about eating, and this time, after you have asked the question, "How hungry am I?" imagine that the number is above a 3, a 5 or 6 for example. Not hungry at all. From this moment on, the first thing you will notice during those times is that since you have become aware of your physical hunger, the sensation of being hungry will subside. You will consciously realize you are not actually hungry.

You may still find yourself wanting something, but at least you understand that it is not hunger. If you do find yourself needing something to satisfy you, you will ask these two simple questions? "What am I feeling right now?" and "What do I need?" Then listen within. Once again, "What am I feeling right now?" "What do I need?" These are the questions you will ask when you come up with a "not hungry" response.

When you get the responses to these questions, your minimum acceptable response is to write them down. Writing them down calms your hunger or craving immediately, because you are giving attention to the real issue at hand. Giving attention to the real issue is the only way you are truly satisfied.

Right now, imagine yourself managing a hunger or craving successfully. First, you will notice yourself wanting to eat something. Next, you stop and ask yourself, "How hungry am I?" You hear your response that you are within the satisfied range, so you then ask, "What am I feeling?" you get a response. Then you ask, "What do I want?" You always get a response. You then write down the answers to "What do I want?" and "What do I need?" You feel happy and satisfied at having managed your craving for food. You simply feel better about yourself.

You recognize the value of this new habit and it is a positive habit that becomes naturally integrated into your life this week and from now on. You are only eating when you are hungry and stopping when you are satisfied.

You are getting in touch with your real needs and are able to fulfill them now that you are writing them down and you are more in touch with how important these other needs are to you. You enjoy working with your body and your hunger scale more and more every day, as it becomes a natural part of your daily routine. You are taking care of your body and respecting the natural wisdom of your mind and your body. You listen to what your body needs and give your body what it wants and deserves. The hunger scale is easy for you to use and you find yourself using it naturally. You are willing to create these new habits permanently in your subconscious mind. Your subconscious mind accepts and receives all these suggestions and they become your reality. Every day in every way you are feeling better and better.

(Trance termination)

Download your scripts at www.VictoriaMGallagher.com/wlpbook

HOMEWORK:

- Listen to recording every day
- Keep an emotional eating journal

Week 3: Visualization

PAPERWORK:

Download Handout at www.VictoriaMGallagher.com/wlpbook

- About Visualization Handout.

FOLLOW-UP FROM LAST WEEK:

- Ask client how many times they listened to their recording.
- Ask client about the emotional eating journal.

Education about Visualization

The first key to getting where you want to be is acknowledging where you are. It's important for you to get some level of acceptance of yourself exactly the way things are right now in your life. Disliking or disowning yourself, your body, or your behaviors usually only makes things worse. There's an old saying that goes, what you resist persists. Meaning, whatever it is about you that you are unwilling to be with and accept, you only attract more of it to be in your presence by resisting it or rejecting it. Of course, many people fear that if they accept their problem, they will keep it or that they are giving up on themselves. Quite to the contrary. Accepting the problem will help you to overcome it much faster than you ever thought.

In this next session, I invite you to create two screens in your mind. One screen will show your present situation. See all the details as clearly as you can. Experience the present situation with all your senses, see, feel, taste, touch, and smell. You might even feel emotional during this process, which is all the more powerful. You'll surround this screen with a dark frame.

Then on another screen you will experience all the details of your desired outcome. Again, experience as deeply as you can, with all of your senses. This screen you will surround with a light frame.

This is a profound technique and it works beautifully.

Screen of the Mind Script

(Induction)

We will now focus on the image of your body. Begin by imagining a screen out in front of you. It can be any kind of screen you like. A TV screen, a movie screen, a computer screen. What's important is that you use this screen to project images that will run kind of like a movie. Surrounding the screen. Place a black frame. On this screen you will run a movie about your life. The way it is right now. You are playing the leading role in this movie. The movie starts the way ordinary movies start, with the credits. See your name in the credits. With an image of your body the way it is right now.

See the title of this movie as it appears on the screen. It says, "The way it is right now" The movie begins. You will now examine yourself in an objective way... in an accepting way. Before you can truly change something, you realize you must accept the way it is now. While you may want something different for yourself, you cannot move from point A to point B unless you accept that you're at point A. This movie is about point A.

While you're watching this movie, really watch what's happening. Imagine standing in front of a 3-way mirror. You can view your body from every angle. You are completely naked. There is a bright fluorescent light shining on you. It brings out every imperfection about your body. Everything you've ever rejected about this body appears before you. It's o.k. to examine the extra layers of fat surrounding your body.

VISUALIZATION

As you stand there, facing yourself. You begin to notice everything about your body. It's important to really look. When you look at yourself, do you like what you see? How do you feel about this person in the mirror? How do you feel deep down inside? How do you feel about your body?

See your body as the structure through which you experience your life. Allow yourself to notice the discomfort and the heaviness of all the extra weight on your body. Your body is forced to carry all that around. Feel the struggle your body goes through just to make it through the day. How much extra energy is it taking you to get out of bed or to get off the couch or to get in your car every day? What would your body be saying to you if it had its own voice? Notice the expression on your face. See your body the way it is right now. Never again will your body be exactly like this again.

Walk over to the clothes in your closet. Notice different types of clothing. The clothes you can still squeeze into, that feel so uncomfortable. The clothes you've settled for wearing to accommodate your body. The clothes that no longer fit, which you hope you'll fit into again... someday.

Walk over to the kitchen and notice all the food you've overindulged in. What kinds of unhealthy eating behaviors have caused you to gain weight? You may have never admitted these behaviors to anyone before. It's time to be honest, with you. What else is in your movie? Laziness? Excuses? All the reasons... The things you keep telling yourself you'll do about it and haven't. The ways you've denied yourself pleasure to punish yourself for being overweight.

Check in with how you feel right now. Breathe in and notice the feelings that are there and feel them. Let your feelings have their own voice. We expend so much energy trying to hide the feelings that we have. What kind of feelings do you have? Honor yourself and love yourself by honoring any feelings that are there. Examine anything else you want, so you can be free of all the ways this has been limiting you. Release anything you've been holding on to, so you can have what it is you want.

WEEK 3

Now we'll be changing scenes.

First, let's completely erase this old image of yourself from your mind. You can easily do this by creating a relaxing scene. A favorite place. Maybe someplace in nature. Take yourself there now and experience yourself enjoying this place for a few moments...

Imagine another screen out in front of you. Surround this screen with beautiful white light. Radiant white light... The light around this screen is so white, you see little flecks of all the colors that make up that white light. You will now run the new movie exactly the way you would have your life be if you could have anything you desire.

Again, you have the leading role in this movie. The movie begins with the credits and once again your name appears. You see an image of yourself. The title of this movie is "What I desire to create in my life right now."

The movie begins. As you once again see an image of yourself in a three-way mirror. You notice something is dramatically different. As you stand there before yourself, completely naked, you give all of your attention to every detail of your body. Look at it closely. See it as an ideal body image. See it as the body you know you can achieve.

It's normal and natural for your body to be firm, strong, and healthy. Notice the reflection, starting from your toes, and slowly moving upward toward your head. Examine every element of this beautiful body. This work of art, standing majestically before you... Notice the way your legs are sculptured and defined. Bring your stomach into view now. Become aware of the way your stomach is flat and firm.

Visualize how your chest area is formed just right, exactly the way you like it. Allow your arms to come into focus. Your arms are strong with exactly the right amount of muscle. Feel your body as it stands before you. You stand straight, tall, and proud. See your face in the mirror. Notice a healthy happy person standing there. See yourself smiling.

You completely honor and respect your body. It feels completely natural to enjoy doing healthy things for your body. You're sensing a renewed feeling of love for this body of yours. A feeling of pride... You have a newfound willingness to treat this body the way it deserves to be treated. You have a sense of appreciation for your body. This body is your best friend.

Now put a picture of the behaviors you want to create on the screen out in front of you. I'll continue giving you suggestions while you imagine yourself behaving exactly the way you prefer from this point forward. Notice the food choices you're making now. Your body deserves and craves healthy foods. Healthy, lean, wholesome, and nutritious foods... Your body craves nutrients, like the ones found in fruits, vegetables. You feel compelled to choose these kinds of foods. Your body craves nutrients found in lean meats. You have a desire to feed your body only the types of food that will enhance your body. You are making sensible, conscious food choices.

Water has become increasingly more attractive to you. Your body craves water. Water has become an important part of your lifestyle. You understand the cleansing affect that water has on your physical body. Your body needs an enormous amount of water. Pure water has a new meaning to you. Being kind to your body means giving it lots and lots of fresh water throughout each day.

You have a strong desire to keep your body in motion. You enjoy the energy that comes with exercising. You enjoy the way stretching your muscles out, releases the toxins from your muscles. You look forward to the tingling sensation of stretching because you know that it's doing your body good. You look forward to the warm burning sensation you get from exercising the muscles in your body. You love the way it feels to breathe deeply and have a routine to help you focus on your breathing on a regular basis. Exercising is an enjoyable part of your day. You exercise regularly. You work on sculpting your body in a way that is pleasing for you and others to look at. You enjoy the energy that exercise gives you.

Your body is your best friend. You enjoy being a friend to your body. From now on listen to what your body wants. From now on, you give your body what your body needs. From now on you protect and honor your body.

(Trance termination)

Download your scripts at www.VictoriaMGallagher.com/wlpbook

HOMEWORK:

- Listen to this recording every day
- Bring affirmation poster to next session.
- Review About Visualization handout.

Week 4: Access the Cause

PAPERWORK:

Download Forms at www.VictoriaMGallagher.com/wlpbook

- Weight Loss Questionnaire

FOLLOW-UP FROM LAST WEEK:

- How many times did they listen to their recording?
- Did they remember to bring their affirmation poster?

Education about Regression

This week we are going to use a technique called hypnotic regression. Regression will help you to recall experiences from an earlier time in your life that may have been responsible for creating the issue you are dealing with today. Going back to that time is a way for you to understand the cause of your problems in such a way that you can easily transform those old beliefs into whatever you would want them to be. Knowing what these old outmoded beliefs are that you are carrying around can be powerful and transformative in and of itself.

Going into regression takes practice, which is why we are not doing this until week 4. It requires a certain level of trust and honesty. I trust that by now you have done all your hypnosis sessions up to this point and that going into hypnosis is something you can do rather easily now.

When you are in regression, you will be able to recall moments in your life you may have forgotten about. You may experience these events happening as if you were right there in the scene. Or, you may experience it like you are remembering something.

Whatever way you experience it for yourself is how you are supposed to experience it. The memories may sometimes not make any sense to you. Follow them anyway. They may be leading you to something that will make sense. You will never actually leave this present moment in time. You will always be fully aware of the fact that what you are experiencing is simply a memory and you can come back to the present moment any time you wish. The best way to understand hypnotic regression is to do it a couple of times.

There may be several experiences or times in your life causing you to keep the weight on. I recommend working with one cause at a time.

The recording we'll be making during today's session will help guide you back into times in your past where you may have learned to hold on to weight. Each time you regress back, you can clear a new issue, or work on any unresolved issues which you may not feel complete on.

If and when you find yourself unable to recall anything else that feels significant to you, then you can stop listening to this recording and play one of your other recordings instead.

Now that I've given you a brief understanding of what to expect, let's go ahead and get started.

Access the Cause Script

(Induction)

In a moment you are going to allow your subconscious mind to become aware of some of your earliest memories, seeking out those things that have caused you to gain weight.

Right now, you may not remember or be in touch with anything that has caused this, or you may be in touch with some of those inner truths already or they may be beginning to surface, as you continue to go deeper into this trance.

In either case, I'm going to be deepening your level of trance in such a way that you' will allow yourself to go back and view the earliest memories of the primary cause of this problem with your weight. Those memories will be there in your vivid memory and be available for you to understand in a new way, with new understandings so that you can release them and become free of all the ways they have limited you.

You will experience that time in your past that holds the cause of your current issue with your weight. You will always be able to view these experiences from a higher perspective.

Your subconscious mind holds every memory you have ever experienced. Your subconscious mind knows exactly how to locate that thing in your past that is causing this problem with your weight. Your subconscious mind will go back to that moment in time when you first experienced this problem at the count of three. At the count of three, you will be vividly in touch with all that you were feeling, experiencing, and thinking back then. Let's begin.

#1... Going back in time... feeling yourself effortlessly floating back to the first time you have ever experienced anything having to do with this problem.

#2... That's right, the information you need will be there for your use, like going to a library, checking in the reference section and having all that information right there at your fingertips so that you can resolve this issue for good.

#3... you are remembering a situation, whatever that situation is. Allow yourself to explore that situation easily and effortlessly and I'll give you a moment to do that now.

(Pause one minute)

Good, now whatever is in your scene, observe all of the details of the scene. Work with whatever senses seem more available to you... maybe you notice physical sensations in your body... experience that feeling fully as if you were right there in that moment. Maybe it was an emotion you felt. Feel the feeling as if you were right there, right now. Maybe there are things that are being spoken to you, your own thoughts or someone else's words. Experience this as best as you can with all of your senses. I'll be silent again so you can take a moment to connect with yourself at this point in time.

(Pause one minute)

That situation has become clearer to you. Can you see how this has created this problem for you today? Then at this point, Invite your adult self into this scene. Since this time in your life you have developed new understandings and wisdom. I'd like this part of you to come into this scene and have a voice, to speak to your younger self during that moment you are still experiencing now and share a new understanding. I'll give you some quiet time to do this.

(Pause one minute)

Very good. You have a new resource of information in the same place in your mind where this past conditioning is stored. Now, re-experience yourself back in that old scene. However, this time, you will re-run the scene as yourself then, with the new understandings... See yourself in that old scene as a transformed person, acting and behaving with these new understandings as if you had known this all along. Sense in some way that a transformation is taking place in your cells, creating new memory, new wisdom.

At this point in time, while you are still in that past situation, when I count to 3, while remaining in a hypnotic state, open your eyes and read your positive suggestions. I will give you a few moments of silence to allow you to let the suggestions sink in. If you have all ten of your suggestions memorized and feel like you would rather do this with your eyes closed that would be fine too. You simply bypass the next suggestions for opening and closing your eyes. On the count of three, you will open your eyes. You will feel slightly out of it and groggy, but you will be aware enough to receive and accept the suggestions you have written down for yourself. 1. 2. 3. Open your eyes and read your suggestions.

(Pause one minute)

Good, you can set that aside and let go and rest back into a deep hypnotic state. Good and go deeper now. Every time you hear me mention the word deeper you will feel yourself resting even deeper than before. Go deeper. Good. Resting ever so deeply. Deeper. You are changing your life for good and permanently. Your new suggestions are implanting themselves on every cell of your body and creating the wonderful positive benefits you want them to create.

Good. Allow that old problem to be completely healed and resolved. If there is any reason it is not already resolved, allow the part of you that is still there to become known to you so it can be released and healed in your next session. Each and every time you do this, you will resolve it more and more completely.

Now allow yourself to gently let go of that old experience completely. Bring yourself back into the present moment in time. Take a moment to understand all that has just taken place. Breathe in these new understandings and breathe out any old recollections of how things used to be. Let go of those old memories completely. Trust that you have done everything correctly and that everything you want to have happen, will happen for your benefit and your highest good, which means the highest good of all beings.

(Trance termination)

Download your scripts at www.VictoriaMGallagher.com/wlpbook

HOMEWORK:

- Listen to this recording every day

Week 5: Drink Water

PAPERWORK:

Download Forms and Handouts at www.VictoriaMGallagher.com/wlpbook

- Article about Water
- Water Drinking Weekly Journal

FOLLOW-UP FROM LAST WEEK:

- How many times did they listen to their recording?

Education about Drinking Water

Note to therapist: I strongly recommend reading and having your client read the book: "Your bodies many cries for water" by Fereydoon Batmanghelidj, M.D. which you will find on Amazon.com.

Drinking water is one of the most important habits you can ever create for yourself. Not only will water help you to reduce weight. It will help you with a wide range of other ailments, including stress, depression, fatigue, allergies, arthritis, and digestion problems to name a few.

By instilling this simple habit of drinking water, you are not only doing something wonderful for your body, but you are increasing your self-confidence.

They say the ideal amount of water to drink is 8 glasses or 64 oz per day. That may work for some. However, our bodies are not all the same and some people require more water. One way to measure the right amount of water for your body is by your weight. Divide your weight in half and whatever number you come up with is the amount of oz of water you should be drinking daily. Spread your water drinking throughout the day to get the most benefit from it.

We're going into hypnosis to cause you to want to drink more water. One last thing, if you are already drinking enough water, listening to this program will still benefit you because it's going to cause the water to have a new effect on your body.

Drink Water Script:

(Induction)

Now you're in a sleep like state, where your subconscious mind is open and receptive to all of the suggestions, I'm about to give you. That's right. let yourself relax and float and drift in this wonderful hypnotic state. Good. You're enjoying this restful peace... This feeling, this wonderful restful relaxation feels so good... so wonderful.

You feel inside of yourself a sense of self-love growing. That's right. Allow that feeling to grow and expand. Feel that deep sense of self-appreciation and gratitude you have for yourself. Realize all of the accomplishments you're so proud of having completed in your life. That's right.

Look at all of the things you have done and achieved for yourself and for other people. Bring to mind all the joy you have brought to other people during your life. You're now able to bring that same joy to yourself. You're able to bring that out and allow that joy to create a new positive healthy you. Where you feel in control.

You feel alive and wonderful in such a way that you want to eat proper foods. Nurturing you. Nurturing yourself by giving your body and all the cells in your body all the water that it needs, loves, wants, and requires to function in a healthy manner. That's right. You are nurturing you. Giving yourself that love every time you drink a glass of water.

You're feeling that love welling up inside of yourself. Knowing you're doing a wonderful thing for your body. You feel so good. That causes you to feel so peaceful and content. If there are any emotions you have about this right now, just bring those up. That's right. Those feelings want to be expressed. They've wanted to be expressed for a long time.

Know you can feel so good sometimes that it can almost feel like pain. When that happens, it may even cause tears to come to the surface and that's o.k. Yes, allow any feelings you have positive or negative to all come up to the surface to be experienced right now. That's good.

You're doing a wonderful job. While you're in this state, allow my words to echo through you. You allow yourself in your inner mind to hear these words over and over.

I deserve to give my body what it loves and what it wants. My body deserves to be taken care of properly. That's right. Say it again. My body deserves to be nurtured and taken care of properly and I do love myself. I do the things that cause me to feel so good. I take care of myself.

I choose to eat the right kinds of food. Craving the kinds of food like raw fresh vegetables. When you think of raw fresh vegetables, you think of them in a new way now. You think of them for how healthy and delicious and crisp they are. You think about all the nutrients that go into your body, to nurture your body. That's right. You think of them in a new way.

Whenever you think about the carbohydrates you used to eat, you realize you don't have a need for them at all. What you're craving is nutritious healthy whole foods. Real foods. Real natural foods make you feel so good about yourself.

We're going to talk about water for a moment. Water has been used for many years to heal all kinds of health conditions. Water is also used in helping people to reduce weight. Water has been one of the best-kept secrets used to reduce weight from your body. You realize this and you now desire to take advantage of all the many benefits drinking water has in store for you.

One of the reasons why water is used to reduce weight is because sometimes your body may have had a tendency to hold on to water. When you don't drink enough water, your body thinks it is in a drought. The more water you drink, the more water you release.

The more water you drink, the more water you crave as well as all the good healthy foods you like in the right amounts. That's right, you turn to smaller portions of food since you have been drinking enough water and you have enough water in your system.

You are now feeling full and satisfied having smaller portions of food. You have that love inside of yourself and that nurturing and caring feeling for yourself, that is causing you to feel full and satisfied, with smaller portions of food.

Imagine yourself, reaching for foods that are low in fat and feeling full and satisfied after eating an amount that you know is appropriate. Whatever amount that might be. You know what's appropriate. The more water you drink, the more you feel full and satisfied. You feel you can do this. You are doing something for yourself that shows your body that you care about it.

Drinking water is something that causes you to feel self-love. This is the way you'll feel each time you have a glass of water, and you'll have many throughout the day. You'll have many glasses of water throughout the day. Each time you take that glass of water; see that glass of water in a new way from now on. See that water as love pouring into your body. That's right. Pouring in love. Sending that love throughout your body and that love radiates throughout your entire being.

Each and every time you pick up and drink that glass of water, that is an opportunity to give yourself some love. That's right. Each and every time you have that glass of water; you're going to remember these good, loving feelings. These wonderful good feelings about your pride, and all of the things you have accomplished in your life.

You will focus on all of the wonderful things that are going on in your life right now and all of the wonderful future accomplishments you will soon have. That's right. Every time you drink a glass of water, (and you do look forward to each and every glass of water you drink), each and every time you get to feel these feelings, these wonderful feelings of self-love, nurturing, coming into your body. That alone causes you to feel full and satisfied. It causes you to want to only reach for foods that would nurture and support this wonderful body of yours.

Some of the benefits you're noticing now as you're taking care of your body, you're healing... You're noticing a healing and renewing taking place in all of your bodily functions. Reducing your cholesterol level and your blood pressure. You're looking better. You're wearing your clothes the way you like to wear your clothes. Feeling so wonderful and so proud of yourself. That's right and that feels so good.

You love the benefits of water. You can drink other things as well, but now you know that each time you drink a soda or something other than water, you will drink one additional glass of water to replenish the dehydrating chemicals contained in coffee, sodas, teas, or alcoholic beverages.

You look forward to drinking more and more water. The more water you drink, the more opportunity there is for you to feel this self-care and self-nurturing. Water is the key here. Water triggers that feeling of self-love. Consider it as a tool for loving yourself. Consider it as a key.

Water invigorates you; it energizes you, and causes you to feel so good, so invigorated, so much energy that you feel motivated to exercise. You know your body wants it.

Now imagine yourself exercising. Imagine all those wonderful positive feelings you have coming in. Notice all the energy that exercise gives to you. That's right you're taking time for you, taking time to nurture your soul, and this body of yours, loving yourself. Those same wonderful positive feelings you have while you're drinking water; you get to experience those same wonderful feelings every time you exercise. You're finding yourself looking forward to those activities. You can hardly wait. You want to exercise. You want to exercise because it causes you to feel so good.

Your day is incomplete without having all the water; at least 8 glasses or 64 oz a day and your day is incomplete without at least a few minutes of exercise. Even if you spent 30 seconds exercising, that will be enough. What you're going to find is that even though you say you're only going to spend 30 seconds exercising, you find the pleasure it gives you, the feeling, welling up, inside your heart, feelings of love, feelings of invigorating energy running throughout your entire body, are going to cause you to want to exercise a little longer than that. However long is up to you.

The key is the water, the exercise, and the self-love... All of that is causing you to eat less, eat smaller portions. You even fill yourself up by listening to this hypnosis program each and every day.

That's another area that we want to focus on is listening to this program, each and every day. That is something you love to do. You love to take this time for yourself because it makes you feel so good. You remember that any time that there's a moment where you feel like maybe you want to sit down and have something to eat. The first thing you're going to think is this, "Have I listened to my hypnosis today?" And if the answer is no then you will decide right then and there to listen to your hypnosis. That is what you'll choose to do.

You are in control. You decide when it's time to eat. You decide when you want to feel good and when you want to feel the love. You choose to feel all those wonderful nurturing feelings you experience when you do hypnosis. Not a day goes by without doing hypnosis. Not a day goes by without doing hypnosis. Every single day, it is the most important thing you have to do all day.

Even if you're not aware of it, these suggestions are going into your subconscious mind and they are supporting you and you know that. You know that these suggestions are going deep into your subconscious mind every day. You're feeling better and better about yourself from a place way deep inside. That is causing the weight to come off. That is causing you to make the right food choices for your health.

DRINK WATER

Your health is most important in your life right now. That is your top priority. This is how you love yourself. That is how you nurture yourself. That's how you get what you need from yourself, from deep inside of you.

You're feeling that pure love, flowing inside of yourself. Feeling proud of you. Feeling successful and being able to control your health, being able to control what you eat. Being in control of your health makes you feel proud. Taking the time for you and to enjoy you. You deserve to feel good about yourself. That's right. You really do like you. You know what it feels like to be thin and in control.

You're beginning, beginning right now, to start to feel that way again. Each and every day that feeling grows a little more. You're more in control each and every day. It's growing more and more. You're feeling so proud. Feeling so successful. You know that this is the most important thing in your life.

Once again, water is the key here. Water is the trigger that is going to trigger that emotion. Trigger the feeling of self-love and that self-love is going to fill you up. That self-love is going to cause you to feel full and satisfied. That's right. With an appropriate, healthy, level of food. Drinking that water triggers that need to want to take even better care of you. Wanting to nurture you by getting plenty of rest and plenty of exercise.

All of these feelings continue to grow and grow inside of you. Your body is shrinking... shrinking and releasing. Releasing water, releasing fat, releasing weight. Releasing it for good so that you free yourself of it forever. That's right. Release it.

Continue to release it until you reach your ideal weight, your goal weight. At that point, you'll move onto a maintenance program. You'll continue eating and exercising in just the right amount to maintain your healthy weight.

Knowing the light and the love, that place inside of you is expanding and your body is shrinking, releasing and letting go. Shrinking, letting go. Release. Release fat. See the fat leaving your body. Let it go. That's right; see it leaving your body. Leaving through drinking an enormous amount of water.

Leaving through sweating during your exercise, and even releasing while you're sleeping.

That's right, you let it go even while you're sleeping. All throughout the night, your body is working toward increasing your metabolism, working on rebuilding your cells, while you're releasing weight. You're doing so good. So now see yourself in whatever way you choose in all future situations with your lean firm healthy body.

(Pause one minute)

Now, each and every time you do this, you allow yourself to imagine yourself in whatever way you want to imagine yourself in your future, laughing, feeling loved, feeling wonderful. You have done so well; you are so proud of yourself and feel so successful. That's right, each and every time you listen to this program, you're going to let those suggestions come in even deeper.

You are awakening to that sense of self-love and that you can do this. That's right you know that it is possible. This can happen for you. You know, you are taking back control of your weight. That's right, taking it back. You are in control.

(Trance termination)

Download your scripts at www.VictoriaMGallagher.com/wlpbook

HOMEWORK:

- Listen to recording every day
- Keep a daily journal of how much water they drink

Week 6: Exercise

PAPERWORK:

Download Forms and Handouts at www.VictoriaMGallagher.com/wlpbook

- Article about Exercise
- Simple Exercise Journal

FOLLOW-UP FROM LAST WEEK:

- How many times did they listen to their recording?
- How much water did they drink?

Education about Exercise

Note to therapist: Suggested reading: Body for Life http://www.bodyforlife.com

This week we will add exercise to your program. Now that we have laid down some of the fundamentals and created some new habits, we're going to help you to increase your motivation and drive to exercise.

Exercise will help you to increase your energy. It will help you to raise your resting metabolism, which causes you to burn more calories throughout the day. When you exercise, you will feel like you want to eat healthier foods. You put an end to cravings for foods with high sugar content since you receive the same effect you get from a sugar rush, through a more natural means called an endorphin rush. You crave more water.

The health benefits I could mention about exercise are simply endless. Whether you exercise for 30 seconds a day or an hour per day, this week we want to get you in the habit of exercising on a regular basis.

Exercise Script

(Induction)

You now desire to create a lean firm healthy body. Your subconscious mind is hearing and receiving everything I'm telling you. Everything I'm telling you begins working immediately. Everything continues to work automatically after you awaken. You won't need to consciously remember anything I tell you. All you need to do is relax.

To reduce your body and develop a strong slender healthy firm body, your subconscious mind is causing you to automatically make proper changes in your eating habits...your subconscious mind is causing you to automatically make proper changes in your eating habits...your subconscious mind is causing you to automatically make proper changes in your eating habits.

It's causing you to exercise your body properly, in ways that are easy and enjoyable to you. That's right... your subconscious mind is causing you to exercise your body properly, in ways that are easy and enjoyable to you. Your subconscious mind is causing you to exercise your body properly, in ways that are easy and enjoyable to you. In ways that make you feel good. In ways that make you feel toned. In ways that give you a sense of accomplishment.

Exercise makes you feel so good. Exercise makes you feel good. Exercise makes you feel good. Exercise makes you feel good. Exercise makes you feel toned. Exercise makes you feel toned. Exercise makes you feel toned.

You notice a sense of accomplishment every time you exercise. You enjoy that sense of accomplishment. You feel yourself become younger and you have more energy to do what's important to you. You feel like you want to accomplish more. You feel like you are ready for the day.

Any obstacles that used to prevent you from exercise are now gone and they are becoming a part of your past. You now find exercise much more important. You imagine yourself getting ready for your workout, however you want to see yourself doing it. Whether it's the first thing you do when you wake up, or on your way home from work, whether you go to a gym, go for a walk, or doing some other activity like hiking, or swimming, or yoga. There is some exercise and some time of day that your body knows works best for you. You allow that image of yourself preparing for doing that activity at that particular time to form in your mind right now. Notice what time it is. Notice what clothes you're putting on to prepare for your workout. See yourself in your work out. I will give you a moment to visualize this now.

(Pause one minute)

Before you go to bed each evening, you will replay that scene you've created, and you will fall asleep with this image of yourself exercising in your mind. You'll repeat that image like a movie several times each night before falling asleep. You notice when you wake up, you have an ever-increasing desire to recreate these events the same way you imagined the night before. Then you will follow through by exercising in reality. Just the way you imagined. Putting on your clothes, noticing that even the time you imagined on the clock is exactly how you envisioned it.

Exercise is good for your health. It helps you to regulate your appetite. Exercise causes you to desire only foods that are beneficial to your body. Exercise causes you to feel content and completely satisfied, when you've eaten exactly the amount of food your body needs to keep you healthy and slender.

You enjoy exercise. You do enjoy exercise. You enjoy exercise. You feel balanced and strong. You feel balanced and strong. You notice you are reducing your body and your body is becoming healthier and firm. You find that it causes your body to feel and look more youthful. Doing exercise regularly is causing your circulatory system to function properly. Doing exercise regularly is strengthening your blood vessels, permitting the blood to flow through every part of your system, strengthening your heart.

You feel good about exercising because it's strengthening your bones. Exercise causes your skin to be firm and smooth. It enables you to sleep more peacefully and comfortably when you go to bed to sleep. You awaken each morning feeling rested and refreshed.

You continue to move into a deeper more peaceful hypnotic state now. Your subconscious mind understands that I'm telling you only things you know you can do, and you enjoy doing everything I'm telling you. You enjoy following an exercise routine and having control over what you eat because it enables you to easily reduce your body and get rid of any excess skin, lumps, or fat. Your entire body becomes firmer.

You understand your body is becoming stronger and firm in an easy and natural way. Your subconscious mind understands everything I'm telling you and is causing your body to function properly.

You are automatically eliminating excess weight from your body. You are automatically eliminating excess weight from your body. You are automatically eliminating excess weight from your body.

You are thrilled to notice your body becoming firm and youthful looking. It's normal for your body to be firm. It's natural for your skin to be firm, smooth, and healthy. Your digestive system, your assimilation system, your metabolism, and your elimination system know how to function perfectly.

It is normal for your body to be slim and firm and trim. In fact, everything I'm telling you is normal for your body. Everything I'm telling you is a part of your real nature. Your subconscious mind is receiving everything I tell you and is causing it to be used effectively for you.

You are drinking a lot of water each day. Water is good for your body. Water is good for your body in all kinds of ways. You have a strong desire to reduce your body.

Your own determination is causing your willpower and self-control to keep increasing. Your own determination is causing your willpower and self-control to keep increasing. Your own determination is causing your willpower and self-control to keep increasing.

Your subconscious mind is cooperating by causing you to select only foods that are needed to keep your body strong, healthy, and slender. You eat only when your body needs food.

You are beginning to feel content more and more each day. You are feeling enthusiastic. You are feeling happy and excited. You sense a feeling of satisfaction from putting everything I tell you into your own actions, knowing it is your own accomplishment. You enjoy doing something every day that's helping your body to continue reducing weight. What you do will be your own accomplishment and will bring you an abundance of feelings of happiness, joy, and accomplishment. Every day you enjoy the wonderful feeling of knowing you are achieving your goal.

(Trance termination)

Download your scripts at www.VictoriaMGallagher.com/wlpbook

HOMEWORK:

- Listen to recording every day
- Write or find an exercise routine that they would like to implement and bring a copy to next hypnosis session.
- Do a minimum of 30 seconds of exercise every day.

Week 7: Eat Healthy

PAPERWORK:

Download Forms and Handouts at www.VictoriaMGallagher.com/wlpbook

- Nutrition handout
- Healthy Eating Plan

FOLLOW-UP FROM LAST WEEK

- How many times did they listen to their recording?
- Talk about the exercise routine

Education about Healthy Eating:

We are now half-way through the program. Let's check in with a few of the habits you have incorporated since the program began. This would be a great point in time to note where you are having the most success and where you may need a little extra support. Once we have gone through the entire program, we can always go back and brush up on any of the programs you would like to strengthen.

- Do you look over your affirmation poster every day?
- How about your hunger scale? Are you using that tool?
- Water drinking? Have you been increasing your water consumption?
- And how about exercise?

Now on to healthy eating. This week the focus will be for you to learn about different foods and eating programs and to choose something you can stick with. In this hypnosis program, the focus will be around a regular balanced diet, reinforcing specific eating behaviors you will want to acquire at this point. If you have a particular diet you like to follow that is different from the nutritional standards presented here, simply substitute whatever words and pictures work best for you.

Eat Healthy Script

(Induction)

This week we will be creating some new messages about healthy foods and healthy eating. Let's begin by imagining all the foods that you used to enjoy that have been giving you a problem. Imagine you are placing all of those old destructive foods that are responsible for putting fat on your body, on a cloud out in front of you. All those greasy, fatty foods, snack foods, junk foods, excessively sweet foods, take them all and put them on that cloud out in front of you. Notice them all piled up on top of one another on that cloud and how heavy and distasteful they look. Notice how they are becoming more and more distasteful looking. Notice the grease and all the fat on those foods, dribbling over the sides. Quickly notice areas of your body where all that fat from those foods was being stored.

Go back to the cloud with all that food on it and give it a push and watch it float away. Bye-bye. Watch closely so you can see it get smaller and smaller and disappear out of existence and out of your life for good. They are gone now, and you forgotten how those foods taste or smell now or even the look of some of those old destructive foods.

You are discovering in their place all of the wonderful, healthy foods your body enjoys as you become trim and slender and reduce your body to your ideal weight. You remember that you enjoy eating foods like lean meats, poultry, fish, fruits, and vegetables. You are discovering a sense of freedom from eating sweets and greasy fattening foods.

Every day your desire for healthy foods is greater than your desire for unhealthy foods. You notice you get much more energy and enjoyment from eating crisp wholesome vegetables. You enjoy savoring the wonderful flavor you get from lean meats. At breakfast time, which is an important time to eat, you enjoy biting into your favorite fresh fruit, nature's dessert.

You enjoy eating small portions, which allows you to eat more often throughout the day and is the best way to increase your metabolism. Notice how your body is becoming lean in those places where there used to be fat. Notice how when you put lean foods into your body, your body becomes lean.

You'll now create in your mind, a list of all the healthy foods you know are appropriate for you. Write them down in any order you like. I'll give you a moment to do that. Keep in mind your body needs over forty nutrients for optimum health. Plan on a wide variety of food and a wide variety of nutrients.

(Pause one minute)

Good.

Imagine yourself taking that list to the grocery store, or wherever you might shop for food, and see yourself going through the store and picking out those foods and checking them off your list. You're picking out foods that give you plenty of protein, like low-fat meats and dairy products, reading the labels and choosing items that have ingredients you know are healthy for you to consume.

You are picking out your fruits and vegetables. These kinds of foods provide the valuable fiber and vitamins your body craves. Fruits and vegetables are filling and satisfying and give you a good sense of well-being. Eating lots of fresh fruits and vegetables is good for your peace of mind. These are your power foods. These foods have fiber, vitamins, minerals and nutrients that are antioxidants for your body, protect your body, and improve your immune system.

You choose to increase your fiber intake through foods like pears, strawberries, avocado, apples, raspberries and other

WEEK 7

high-fiber fruits. You choose to increase your fiber intake through foods like broccoli, brussels sprouts and other high-fiber vegetables. You choose to increase your fiber intake through foods like lentils, kidney beans, split peas, chickpeas, and other high fiber legumes. You choose to increase your fiber intake through foods like quinoa, oats, and other high-fiber grains. You choose to increase your fiber-intake through high-fiber nuts and seeds.

It simply makes you feel good to eat these positive healthy foods. These are foods you were meant to eat. These foods are sensible and help you to reduce your body to the level you want it to be and maintain it.

Now that you have finished your shopping, imagine yourself in your daily routine, in the morning, waking up having whatever you will have at breakfast time. Remember to eat slowly, taking small bites. Enjoy the color, the taste and the texture of your food.

Remember it takes 20 minutes before that satisfied feeling registers.

Good. You are now having a mid-morning snack. You are concentrating only on eating when you eat. You enjoy eating as a single-focused activity and you now notice the flavor of your food, which helps you to become satisfied with a small portion.

It's now lunch time and you are enjoying a meal again. Notice how you enjoy getting to eat this often and only a small portion. This way of eating is helping you to increase your metabolism.

It's now time for your mid-afternoon snack. Remembering to eat a small amount of these healthy foods, getting in the habit of eating 5 times a day, these positive power foods.

Moving on to dinner time. You notice you are able to eat calmly. Good. Notice how wonderful it feels to spend the day eating only quality foods that are for your quality body. Feeling a sense of peace and pride and confidence in your ability to maintain proper eating habits.

You take control of your healthy eating behavior right now. Each day becomes easy to naturally eat this way. You feel a sense of accomplishment and excitement because you know you are doing a good thing for your body. You do realize now more than ever that you enjoy eating healthy each day. You enjoy the health benefits you are receiving from eating healthy. It makes you feel good. It gives you energy. It keeps you looking good, looking younger.

You are seeing the results in your body, becoming leaner all the time. It helps you to create a more positive attitude about yourself and about life in general. You want only these kinds of foods from now on because you know they are doing your body good. Your body is becoming more fit and beautiful and pure and natural every day. You feel good about your commitment to yourself and you do your best every day. You love and respect your body. Good.

(Trance termination)

Download your scripts at www.VictoriaMGallagher.com/wlpbook

HOMEWORK:

- Create a healthy eating plan and bring copy to next hypnosis session.
- Listen to recording every day
- Eat according to the new healthy eating plan at least 5 days this week.

Week 8: Metabolism

FOLLOW-UP FROM LAST WEEK:

- How many times did you listen to the recording?
- Discuss new healthy eating plan?
- How many times did you eat according to the new eating plan?

Education about Metabolism

Let's spend a moment now getting acquainted with the process in your body called your metabolism. Your metabolism is the part of you that is responsible for burning calories. Calories are just another word for energy. Your body is in constant need of energy and therefore calories are being burned all day long no matter what you are doing, running, walking, eating, sitting, and even while you are sleeping. This is all a function of your metabolism.

A couple of the normal ways your metabolism becomes activated to turn up the volume of its calorie burning routine are when you eat and when you exercise. This is called a thermogenic response. Thermogenic response means heat production. Heat production means your body's temperature rises, which in turn burns fat.

One of the ways your metabolism is affected is based on the way your body is composed of fat and muscle. The more muscle you have the more energy you need to maintain those muscles. The higher percentage of muscle mass you have, the more energy your body has to burn, i.e. the higher your metabolism.

WEEK 8

Another element to being able to increase your metabolism is oxygen. We're going to do a series of deep breathing exercises and visualizations now to cause your body to increase your resting metabolism.

Metabolism Script

(Induction)

As you are lying there resting, your subconscious mind will remember the process we are going to do and cause your body to make the proper changes associated with increasing your metabolism. Just lay with your body completely still and peaceful.

Imagine an energy that is emanating from within your body. Imagine it is a white light or maybe a light that has a golden glow to it. Imagine you are looking at the energy running through the inside of your body. You may even feel the tingle of that glow as you place your attention on any particular area of your body.

Good ... as you look even closer at that energy you see that there is a vibration. That energy vibrates and moves through your body and touches every cell, every bone, every organ, and every tissue. It runs through your body kind of like a river.

While you pay vivid attention to this energy running through your body, take in a slow and deep breath way down deep into your belly. Pay particular attention to that energy as you slowly take in that breath. Do that a few times until you notice something different about that energy. You now realize you have complete control over what that energy does. You can change the quality of that that energy. You may notice you want to change the vibration. Maybe it's the glow or the color you'll decide to change.

One thing you notice is that by breathing in this deep and calm way, this energy almost invites more of that wonderful oxygen to become a part of itself. The tiny oxygen molecules blend perfectly with the molecules of your internal energy which is becoming stimulated in some way by that oxygen that you are breathing in and out of your body.

One thing you may have never known before is that oxygen is your key to burning fat from your body. Raising the level of oxygen is your key to raising your metabolism, the rate at which fat is burned from your body. Not only does raising the level of oxygen in your body increase your metabolism, which burns fat from your body, it also helps you to digest your food better.

There are several ways to raise your oxygen level. One of the best ways to increase your oxygen intake is to create a need for it. The more muscle mass you have, the more oxygen your body needs. You may find it desirable to increase your muscle mass by working out with weights. Another way to raise your oxygen level is to eat more often. Eating the right foods more often will help you to raise your metabolism. Of course, we take in oxygen when we breathe, so breathing is a great way to increase your metabolism and increase your energy level.

Again, it's time to breathe, only this time, breathe like this: Inhale through your nose to a slow count of four, breathe in, 2, 3, 4 and hold for 7, 2, 3, 4, 5, 6, 7, and exhale for 8, 2, 3, 4, 5, 6, 7, 8. Good. Let's make sure you got it, breathe in 2, 3, 4, and hold, 2, 3, 4, 5, 6, 7, and release, 2, 3, 4, 5, 6, 7, 8. Good.

Something else you may notice is the temperature in your body increases. Place your attention on your body temperature and notice if you feel slightly warmer than you did before we got started. If you do, good for you, you are already increasing your metabolism by using this visualization. We are going to be doing some more. Let's continue.

Go back to imagine that energy inside your body. We're going to be flexing and releasing different areas in your body, beginning with your toes. If you can do it, continue watching with your mind's eye what is going on inside your body as this is happening. When you flex your feet, you'll do it to the count of your in-breath and while your holding and you'll relax your feet on your out-breath. Ready, flex your toes and breathe in, 2, 3, 4, and hold, 2, 3, 4, 5, 6, 7, and release, 2, 3, 4, 5, 6, 7, 8.

Good. Now your calves, and flex, 2, 3, 4, and hold, 2, 3, 4, 5, 6, 7, and release, 2, 3, 4, 5, 6, 7, 8. Good and your thighs. Flex, 2, 3, 4, and hold, 2, 3, 4, 5, 6, 7, and release, 2, 3, 4, 5, 6, 7, 8. On down to your abdomen and flex, 2, 3, 4, and hold, 2, 3, 4, 5, 6, 7, and release, 2, 3, 4, 5, 6, 7, 8.

You're doing great. Remember your deep breathing and visualize these areas of your body. Moving to your upper arms, ready? Flex, 2, 3, 4, and hold, 2, 3, 4, 5, 6, 7, and release, 2, 3, 4, 5, 6, 7, 8. You'll now make a fist, 2, 3, 4, and hold, 2, 3, 4, 5, 6, 7, and release, 2, 3, 4, 5, 6, 7, 8.

Bring your attention to your face, scrunch up your face and breathe in 2, 3, 4, and hold, 2, 3, 4, 5, 6, 7, and release, 2, 3, 4, 5, 6, 7, 8. Very well. Notice the warm sensation you are creating through your body and check in with the color and the vibration of that energy now. Notice again any changes taking place in the glow and the rate of vibration and understand what those changes mean to you.

We'll now start our journey up the mountain. Imagine yourself at the bottom of the mountain and you are all ready to go. The air around you is crisp and cool. The air is a little thinner when you are in this high altitude, which means you have to breathe deeply. Continue breathing in the pattern we were just doing and begin your climb. As you look up the mountain you can see that it is a pretty steep climb. You are prepared for it. You have everything it takes to get up that mountain. You are breathing properly.

As you imagine yourself on that mountain, you see a person whose muscles are toned and in good shape for a climb. You are following a path straight up the side of that mountain. As you come in contact with any obstacles, you pick them up with full force and toss them out of your way. You feel your muscles working and becoming stronger. You feel the heat in your body burning off layers of fat as you head higher and higher up that mountain.

You are reaching your goal. You feel yourself higher and higher. You notice it does get a little steeper and a little harder to stay committed to your goal of reaching the top of the mountain and you want to stop for a moment but something inside says keep going. Keep going. Keep going.

You are doing excellent. You continue upward. Your muscles are becoming more visible. Your breathing is getting deeper. You become more sensitive to the way your body feels energized or when it's become weighted down with something you don't need. You are able to keep the pace along this mountain path. Look up and see your goal is well within reach. This excites you. Nothing will get in your way of reaching your goal. Your metabolism has reached its full potential. Your body is working optimally.

You feel a sense of pride and victory. You feel like a winner. This motivates you to keep going and continue your progress. You are feeling so healthy. Only a healthy person could achieve such an amazing goal of climbing this mountain the way you have. As you have climbed higher and higher you have raised your metabolism higher and higher to run at an optimum level whether you are resting, eating, or working out.

You are almost there. Only a couple more feet to go and you will have reached your goal. Remember your breathing. Every day you do this exercise, you'll notice new levels of achievement or climb new mountains that you never knew existed before. You'll always get to feel a sense of satisfaction at achieving new levels of accomplishment in your weight and health goals. You'll notice your metabolism functions perfectly and that the control of increasing the level of your metabolism has always resided right within you.

You have the power to do anything you want. You have always had the power. You have reached the top of that mountain and you are feeling the self-confidence and sense of achievement that is just like that feeling of accomplishment you are feeling as you achieve your body's ideal weight, shape, and size. Take a closer look at this person who has just climbed that mountain and see the person who has released all the weight from your body.

As this person comes more and more into focus, listen to anything that you are saying. Feel the way your body feels thin and energetic. It feels good to be in charge of your body, doesn't it? It feels good to be in shape.

Now that you feel so good, go ahead and anchor in this special moment by squeezing your thumb and your forefinger together. Do that now while breathing in the way we've been talking about. Squeeze, and breathe in, 2, 3, 4, and hold, 2, 3, 4, 5, 6, 7, and while keeping your fingers still pressed together, release your breath, 2, 3, 4, 5, 6, 7, and 8.

Good, these lovely feelings have been anchored into your thumb and forefinger, any time you press your thumb and forefinger together, these feelings will come back to you and your metabolism will increase to its optimum level.

You will notice yourself naturally breathing in this new way more and more often, which will greatly improve your metabolism, which is functioning better and better every day, causing your body to burn fat and trim down to the level you desire. Now release your thumb and forefinger and relax and consciously let go of everything you have experienced. Let go for now and I'll give you a few moments of silence to let your mind drift to wherever it wants to go.

(Pause 30 seconds)

Good... press your thumb and forefinger together and notice what is taking place in your body. Feeling all those incredible feelings of accomplishment all right there within you again and if you're not feeling them yet, cause them to be there the way you did before and each time you do this, you will strengthen the effect this anchor has to bring about these incredible feelings much stronger and faster and at any time you wish to call them forth. Release your thumb and forefinger and relax again and let go. Clear your mind completely and rest peacefully.

(Trance termination)

Download your scripts at www.VictoriaMGallagher.com/wlpbook

HOMEWORK:

- Listen to recording every day
- Remember to use your anchor

Week 9: Banish Old Patterns of Behavior for Good

FOLLOW-UP FROM LAST WEEK:

- How many times did you listen to your recording?
- Did you use your anchor?

Education About Swish

During this session you will utilize one of the most powerful techniques of Neuro Linguistic Programming. This particular technique was originated by the famous Psychologist, Richard Bandler, and has since been widely used by students of Tony Robbins books and seminars. It's called "Swish."

Swishing allows you to switch the way you represent things now considered desirable with things you know would be more beneficial. Once you learn how to Swish, you can apply this technique to re-wire your brain to change any habit you desire to change. Before going into this session, what you want to think about is a behavior you would like to change. Be ready with this new behavior change before going into hypnosis.

One thing to note about this technique in particular is you don't have to go deep into hypnosis to do it. All you need is to be able to relax and concentrate on your situation for a few moments. Then, whenever you want to, or you catch yourself about to engage in an undesirable behavior, you can literally do this exercise and get rid of that old habit for good.

Each time you do this, think of a new behavior you'd like to work on. Perhaps one day it's your lack of willpower toward exercise. Another day it could be your desire for sweets. Another day, you might work on being able to get up on time or go to bed on time. Maybe it's being able to maintain a positive attitude throughout the day. Change does not have to take a long time. You can make many changes instantly. As you notice these things working for you, that is something to get excited about.

A final note about visualization. We all have 5 senses, hearing, sight, taste, touch, and smell. The 3 senses that we predominately use to represent things to ourselves are sight, hearing, and feeling. The majority of people are predominantly visual, the next are predominantly auditory, they hear things, and the final group of people are more kinesthetic, feeling people. All of these groups of people overlap in each of those areas. If you are not predominantly visual and you don't get pictures when you do this exercise, part of the reason may be is because you hold a belief that you don't know how to visualize.

However, I'll bet that if I were to ask you to describe where you live or what color your car is or specific visual types of questions, your brain would present you with a quick picture in your mind before you answered my questions. At least this is usually the case. For example, what color is your car? If you said blue or red or whatever, how did you come up with your answer? How do you know it's blue? Are you remembering you bought a blue car and you're hearing the word blue in your mind? Or does your mind quickly flash a picture of your car? Now, you may not be able to hold on to a picture in your mind or see it as close or sharp as you would like. However, this process that we are going to go through is great to remedy that situation. Yes, you can learn how to become more visually oriented. Additionally, you will be working with your other senses. When it comes to the swish part of the technique, maybe you will hear the changing of the frames or you will feel how they do it. You can do this. It just takes a little practice and you will get better at it and be able to create the things you want in your life. Ready? Let's begin.

Swish Script

(Induction)

Now, bring to your mind that behavior you want to change. Get a clear picture of it in your mind. Notice every detail about that scene. Make it as big and bright as possible. In the bottom right-hand corner (and if you're like me, think about where your right hand is before you do this, place a small dark image of the way you would like things to be. Yes, make what you don't want very big and bright and close. Make what you do want tiny small dark and dim. Kind of like the way it is in your life now, right? Alright.

Then, you will take your small picture, in a moment, but not until I say now, and blow it up to the size and brightness of the picture of the behavior you no longer desire. When you do this, which will take you exactly one second of time, you will say the word "whoosh" out loud. Yes, you might feel a little silly saying, "whoosh" out loud, but if that's all it would take for you to become successful, won't you say it?

When I say now, you are going to whoosh that behavior you want right into the same place you are holding that old behavior and you'll do it in one second of time. The image of the thing you don't want will trade places with the thing you do want and be dim and small and down in that right-hand corner. Ready? Do it now. "whoosh"

Good ... Now the new behavior you do want is bright and vivid and close to you. Experience it for a second or two.

(Pause 5 seconds)

Open your eyes so you can clear away that scene completely. Close them again.

Now that you know how to do this, let's do it a little quicker this time. The key to doing this is to do it fast and to do it faster and faster and to do it a number of times. You may lose track of what you are doing consciously and that is perfectly alright because your subconscious mind knows exactly what you are doing and knows how to do it fast, even if you can't consciously keep up with what's happening ok?

Let's reset the scene. This time as you are expanding that picture of the behavior you want to its full size, allow yourself to see, feel, and hear what's happening as that is taking place. Do this even faster than before. Ready? "whoosh"

(Pause 5 seconds)

Good... Give yourself a moment to take in and experience things the way you want them.

(Pause 15 seconds)

Good and now open your eyes and clear your mind. Close your eyes. You know what to do, ready? "whoosh."

(Pause 5 seconds)

Experience it. Wonderful. Open your eyes. Close your eyes, and ... "whoosh" ... stay with it for a little while.

(Pause 15 seconds)

Open your eyes. I'm going to give you a moment to do this over again a few more times, doing it faster and faster each time. Ideally, you want to do this about 5 or 6 times and each series about a 1/2 a second. I'll give you 30 seconds to do the same one over and over and faster and faster. Begin.

(Pause 30 seconds)

Good... Now, how you'll know that this has been successful is that from now on, whenever you see that old image, it will be difficult to see it without this new image being blasted right over it.

You'll now take this new behavior and project yourself into the future. Let's start with tomorrow. What will be happening tomorrow with regard to this new behavior?

As you get these scenes just the way you like them to be, you'll make them brighter and more colorful. Hear them louder. Create the sensations you will feel in your body.

Good... Let's go out to a week from now. What effect is this new behavior having on your life in only one week? What kind of thoughts might you be thinking? What kind of food will you be eating? What kind of activities will you be doing?

Let's now project this behavior out to one month from now. At this time, you see some bigger changes taking place. You might see an image of yourself in the mirror, maybe you're wearing some different clothes. Maybe you are with some friends or family members who are commenting on the results of your new behavior. Maybe it's more energy you notice.

Let's go out to three months from now. What kinds of differences do you notice in only three months? What kinds of emotions do you feel as you recognize the success you have achieved at this point three months from now? You see yourself with the look the represents whatever that emotion may be for you and you bring that image closer, so you can see right into your eyes a glow that is coming from the inside about the incredible changes you have made over this period of time.

Let that time frame become six months from now. Maybe at six months, you still have a sense of excitement about the changes you have made, but at this point in time, the changes have simply become a way of life for you. You feel like a happier person and a successful person and you have a greater sense of gratitude and pride about yourself and your well-being. What else do you notice about yourself?

Moving out to a year from today. What is your life like since you have totally integrated this new behavior into your life? If the person you have become a year from now could tell the person you are in the present moment just one thing, what would they say?

Listen for a response.

(Pause 15 seconds)

Thank your future self for this information now and come back to present time and allow these words of wisdom to become implanted on every cell in your body. These changes in your behavior you desire have already begun to take effect, in the same way that a plant begins to grow the moment the seed has been planted.

Every day the effects of these changes will grow and become stronger and more a part of your reality and you will begin to see evidence of these changes taking place one day, in much the same way that you may not see evidence that there is a plant and then one day, you turn around and you notice that plant sprouted up out of nowhere and suddenly you realize that the seed really did take hold, just like these suggestions are beginning to take hold now.

(Trance termination)

Download your scripts at www.VictoriaMGallagher.com/wlpbook

HOMEWORK:

- Make a list of behaviors they'd like to change – bring to next session.
- Listen to recording working with several of these behaviors over the week.

Week 10: Melt Fat

FOLLOW-UP FROM LAST WEEK:

- Did you bring your list of behaviors?
- How many did you get through?
- How many times did you listen to your recording?

Education about Melting Fat

During this session we're going to take a cellular approach to eliminating fat from your body. Your subconscious mind controls everything, including cell growth. Even when you are doing all the right things for your body, exercising, eating right, relaxing, and getting plenty of water, the fat and the cellulite may have a tendency to hang around longer than you'd like it to. That is because your subconscious mind has a tendency to keep things the same all the time. It's your body's defense mechanism to keep the constancy of things, like blood flow, and temperature running constantly at about the same pace.

Change in physiology can be hard unless you give your subconscious mind new information.

In this program, we will instruct your subconscious mind to create the changes in your physical body you want it to make, reducing and eliminating your fat cells.

Melt Fat Script

(Induction)

You are well on your way to having a slender, firm, toned, and smooth body. Free of bulges... free of lumps... free of cellulite... free of any unnecessary fat. You now eliminate all excess fatty tissue from your body, leaving you with beautiful firm skin and toned muscles, which are sleek and well defined. These changes take effect in every part of your mind and body. These changes take place quickly, effortlessly, and permanently.

You are open and willing to receive these suggestions on every level. Every part of you wants these changes to take place. The guidance and instructions will be firmly implanted at a deep level. Your subconscious mind is ready now and willing to accept every suggestion you allow to create the changes you want to make in your body that are for your benefit and highest good. Every suggestion begins working immediately at the cellular level and your cells respond by causing your body to release any and all impurities. It will form in exactly the way we ask it to.

As these suggestions strongly take hold, you are happy to notice all of that unnecessary cellulite shall cease to exist from your body easily and naturally in the same way you eliminate all waste from your body.

Your body already knows how to do this. In order for your cells to remember how to remove cellulite from your body, let's go over the process of how this will happen. Your subconscious mind controls everything your body does. It causes your heart to beat, your eyes to blink, your breathing, when you're not even thinking about it. It causes the blood to flow.

Your subconscious mind is amazingly powerful the way it keeps track of so much going on inside your body all the time. Your subconscious mind does not work in the same way your conscious mind works... using reason and logic. No, it simply carries out instructions. In much the same way you train an animal to do tricks. You can train your subconscious mind to do some magical things for you and for your benefit.

Your subconscious mind has been trained to do things that are not for your benefit. So now, once your subconscious mind has the new information it will then go right to work and embed and implant the information into your cells which will cause your body to function the way a fit body does as it releases all impurities.

The way your body releases impurities from your body is this: cellulite is made up of liquid, fat, and other waste materials. When the bodily system is not working optimally, an accumulation begins to form as a little pocket under the skin... If it remains in your body, it creates a gel-like substance that shows through the skin looking like a lump or bulge.

The next thing to understand is you already have all the necessary fluids in your body to melt that gel-like substance and transform it into a liquid that is cleansed out of your body easily as you eliminate all waste from your body.

Your subconscious mind is now restoring that system of cleansing and dissolving fat, fluid, cellulite, and other waste from your body to its optimum level of performance.

It's as simple as that. You have been given these instructions at a subconscious level, which will be now carried to every cell in your body so that every cell knows exactly how to respond to the liquids and fats in your body. Your body is extremely intelligent, and it knows exactly how to do this.

From now on, each and every time you drink a glass of water; your subconscious mind will activate the natural fluids in your body so they will liquify any unnecessary lumps or bulges and they will flow along the regular path of eliminating waste from your system.

You are happy to notice your body getting rid of all its unwanted lumps and bulges as the natural fluids and acids in your body are being restored to their proper functioning. Every day you're noticing your body becoming smoother, firmer, and more perfectly developed. Your thighs are becoming smooth and

WEEK 10

firm. Your hips are becoming smooth and firm. Your buttocks are becoming smooth and firm. Your knees and calves are becoming smooth and firm. Your upper arms are becoming smooth and firm. Your stomach is smooth and firm. Your face is smooth and firm. Every day your muscles are becoming more toned as the fat that has surrounded the muscles dissolves. Your skin keeps becoming firmer and you are looking younger.

You love the way your body easily restructures itself perfectly so that it is more ideal for you in its shape and size; exactly the way you desire it to be.

If you listen to this recording every day faithfully, involving yourself emotionally, and working with the visualizations, the improvement will begin to be noticeable to you within the next 7 days. As you keep succeeding at this, the excitement grows, and you will continue to make progress. Keep listening to this program every day and you will be through with all excess cellulite, all excess fat, liquids, and all excess impurities for good.

You will continue to drink water in enjoyable ways. Pure water. Not soda, juice, coffee, tea, or anything else, just water. You drink a minimum of 64 oz of water per day. If you drink any other beverage, you will replace that beverage with an additional 8 oz of water. Any other beverage removes water from your system. You will drink a minimum of 64 oz of pure water every day from now on.

You enjoy making drinking water a part of your life. You enjoy the taste of water. You know that it is helping your body to quickly remove that unsightly cellulite from your body in a new way. Even if the proper amount of water was consumed before, your body now utilizes the water in a new way and that is to wash away all the fat and cellulite out of your body. Wash it away for good.

Drinking water sends a signal to your subconscious mind to turn on the waste elimination process, cleansing your body of all its fat, creating a lean firm, healthy body.

Now ... place your attention on any particular area of your body where you want to remove cellulite immediately. See it exactly the way it is presently. Then ... imagine yourself shrinking down to the size of one of your own cells and going inside your body to that exact place where you have stored cellulite. Create with your imagination, some way to eliminate those fat cells from your body with your vivid imagination. See yourself in there, dissolving those bad cells, or moving them, or blasting them away, in whatever way you wish, getting rid of those fat cells for good.

(Pause one minute)

Good. Now going back out to view the part of your body from the outside and notice how smooth and tone it is. Feel the tightness of your skin. Each time we do this, you focus on that area more, or you can move on to a new area. You will be amazed to notice how powerful your mind really is.

Even though you will notice these changes in your body in about 7 days, these changes will be noticeable to your friends and others within about 14 days as you will be able to wear at least one size smaller than at the beginning of this program. The compliments you receive will help you to continue sticking with this program and reinforce the improvements and progress you are making. Each and every day your body grows stronger, healthier, leaner, in better shape, and trimmer. You feel energized because your body no longer has to lug around those extra pounds of fat.

Every cell of your body is a healthy cell. Each cell creates healthy organs. As your organs continue functioning more perfectly, your body runs more efficiently and more effectively. You want to maintain this healthy body and continue improving all the time in every way. All of the improvements will take a permanent place in your life creating a profound feeling of overall happiness and satisfaction.

(Trance termination)

Download your scripts at www.VictoriaMGallagher.com/wlpbook

HOMEWORK:

- Listen to recording every day

Week 11: Reshape Your Body

FOLLOW-UP FROM LAST WEEK:

- Did you listen to your recording every day?

Education about Reshaping Your Body

This week we are going to work with your body image. You will create a new appreciation for your body and sculpt your body to the image you like it to become. A guide will come to you during your hypnosis session and help you to reshape your body in all the areas.

We can be so hard on our bodies when we are out of shape, hating them, berating them, and even feeling disgusted or embarrassed by them.

We have taken our bodies for granted. Whether you like the image of your body or not, it's been there for you to help you experience your life. As such, this hypnosis session will help you to become a partner with your body and thank it for being here for you. Accepting your body image will help you take a giant step toward changing it.

Note to Hypnotherapist: Toward the end of this session, I mention a 'nurturing and caring soul.' I refer to this being as a 'her.' When working with male clients, adjust the phrasing of the script accordingly.

Reshape Your Body Script

(Induction)

As we begin talking about reshaping your body, the first thing that is important to realize is exactly how this is possible. Your body, which is composed of molecules, enzymes and cells, was designed to function perfectly and healthily.

Being over-weight is unhealthy and is not the way your body was meant to be. The way your body was designed, it is capable of recapturing the form that is normal and natural for your body. It is normal and natural for your body to be slim and trim.

Your body can easily reshape itself as soon as you get a clear image in your mind of exactly the way you would like your body to look. This is true because every cell in your body thinks and every cell is constantly in the process of renewing itself and replacing itself. Your subconscious mind is directing your cells to form in the way you imagine your body in your mind.

During your life, you have imprinted information on your cells to shape your body to the way it is because of the images you created about the way you thought your body should be. These beliefs have been based on the way you identified with your parents' bodies, your relatives, your friends, television, doctors, teachers, and all kinds of other sources. Had you only known you could create an image of how you would want your body to be and hold that image firmly in place, you would have done this long ago.

It's important to appreciate your body exactly the way it is now and that it has served its purpose for you and your body is your friend. It's been carrying this extra weight around for you for years, hasn't it? Believe it or not, your body would rather not have that burden of carrying that extra weight around for you anymore. Every pound off your body will be a welcome relief.

Imagine yourself, having to lug around something that weighs even 10 pounds all day long. Thank your body for being there to carry all that extra weight around. It's time to become partners with this buddy of yours.

Your body can create for you a natural, beautiful, slender, slim, trim, healthy, and strong body. Observe your body, even as it is now as if you were looking through the eyes of a supportive and nurturing friend.

Breathing in slowly and smoothly, gently and easily, taking you down deeper and deeper into relaxation. Feel your body. Become aware of the way your body feels. The way it's positioned. Notice if your body is comfortable in this position and if not, shift your body slightly so you can make it comfortable.

Your treating your body with the utmost care and concern as if you've handed your body over to the most nurturing soul you've ever known and this nurturing and caring soul takes her hands and passes them over your body and you feel a wave of relaxation as her hand passes over each part of your body, creating a warmth and an energy. Your cells respond wonderfully to her touch. You now go deeper into a relaxing hypnotic rest.

Examine your body as it is right now. Examine each area of your body, knowing this is the final time you will see your body exactly like this. Good.

You're going to place your attention on every detail of this body and create it to become exactly the way you want it, ideally as a slender, trim, firm, and toned body that is the real you. Imagine this pleasant nurturing soul standing next to you in a 3-way full-length mirror. You will examine every element of this beautiful body as it stands in front of you. This being will pass her hand over every inch of your body, changing the structure, leaving behind a more sculptured, well-defined and toned body part.

Beginning with your calves, your calves are becoming slender, firm, and trim, shaped exactly the way you like your legs to be.

Her hand moves upward passing over your knees and your thighs. See how your knees and thighs are slim, trim, firm and shaped exactly the way you want your knees and thighs to be.

Now passing over your hips and buttocks, leaving you with slender and firm, perfectly proportioned hips and buttocks.

Her hand passing over your genital area and creating any changes you would like to see in that area.

Her hand is passing over your lower abdomen... your upper abdomen... and your stomach... notice the changes in your mid-section now. You have flat, firm, smooth perfectly developed stomach and abs.

This hand passes over and around your waist area, having a slimming effect, leaving this entire area, your waist, stomach, and abs, completely slender, trim, and firm.

Turning to the back area, these warm, nurturing hands move all around your back area, causing it to form strong and lean back muscles, and correct alignment of your spine so you stand tall and proud.

You turn toward the front again and this hand creates the changes in your chest area to become perfectly proportioned to your body.

This hand passes down your shoulders, your arms and your hands, leaving those areas slim, trim and strong. Back up to your neck and face. Notice when this hand passes over, it leaves a firmness in your neck and your chin and tightens up and lifts the skin on your face so that it is completely smooth and young-looking.

You see your whole body standing before you in that full-length mirror and notice if there are any other areas you would like to change, and you allow that to happen.

An amazing thing happens. You realize this loving, nurturing being who has been doing this wonderful powerful sculpting of your body is you. It gives you a warm and wonderful feeling inside to know you can do something so loving for yourself. You can be so gentle and nurturing and friendly toward your body.

Now that you are standing there next to this ideal body you have created, step inside and see how it feels. Check out every part of your body and if there are parts that you feel you still want to change, allow that to happen. Move around in your body. Feel the strength this body has. Feel the lightness. Notice how good it feels.

Notice, if you haven't already, how natural it feels to be in this body and that these changes are already beginning to take place. This is the body you were meant to have. This is the body you are going to be spending the rest of your life in.

This image of your body makes a firm imprint now on every cell. That's right; scan your whole body to register this image firmly into your subconscious mind. This image becomes an automatic force that reinforces the behaviors and activities in your daily life that support this body.

From this moment forward you will realize an ever-growing respect for your physical body. You realize that in order for your body to be healthy, taking care of your body properly is essential. You realize that in order for your body to do the things you would like it to be able to do; you need to treat your body with respect. You have made a decision to become healthy. You'll be perfectly content with doing healthy things for your body, like giving it proper nutrition, plenty of fresh water, and regular exercise.

You completely honor and respect your body. It feels completely natural to enjoy doing healthy things for your body.

You are sensing a renewed feeling of love for this body of yours. A feeling of pride. You have a newfound willingness to treat this body the way it deserves to be treated.

As you see and feel your whole body, notice your feelings of confidence. These changes have already started, and you will continue to experience these pleasant changes taking place each and every day in every way.

(Trance termination)

Download your scripts at www.VictoriaMGallagher.com/wlpbook

WEEK 11

HOMEWORK:

- Listen to recording every day

Week 12: Maintenance

FOLLOW-UP FROM LAST WEEK:

- Did you listen to your recording every day?

Education about Maintenance

This week will be a recap of all the weeks leading up to today. Acknowledge your client for sticking with the program over these last 12 weeks and any successes that they have achieved.

Remind them that the changes they are making are permanent since we have been working from the inside out.

Suggest that they go over any of the weeks that they need a little refresher on or repeat the program by themselves over the next 12 weeks.

Suggest coming back for monthly follow-ups until their entire goal has been achieved.

Have them listen to this recording you are going to make for maintenance this week and every week until their goal has been achieved, unless they are reviewing other parts of the program.

Maintenance Script

(Induction)

Now that you have come this far, this is only the beginning. You have created extraordinary healthy habits for yourself. You are beginning to realize by the techniques which you have learned over the last several months, lasting change is truly possible.

You know it is. You know it is for you. It's time to give yourself some acknowledgement.

No matter how far you have come, whether it's barely making it through this program, or you have completely achieved your weight goal, you have done some incredible life changing work. It's time now to acknowledge yourself.

Acknowledge yourself for all the success you have achieved at this point in the program. You deserve to be recognized for whatever amount of work went in to getting this far.

Imagine yourself sitting in front of you and letting yourself know how proud you are to have accomplished whatever success you have created for yourself at this point. A few kind words to yourself is all I'm asking you to do. Good.

I'm going to take you back in time. You will be able to remember all the aspects of what you have been through over the past few months. You may have left out some of what has gone into these past 12 weeks.

Let's start back to the day when you searched for this program. You probably went through something that day which made you choose to make a change in your life.

Moving on to the time when you opened the program and you started listening to the introduction and maybe you got a little excited and maybe you still felt skeptical. You continued and you pressed on. You knew some good stuff was going to follow.

You set some goals for yourself, and you created some new affirmations and created posters with those affirmations on them. You began the process of creating a habit of going into hypnosis every day. Acknowledge yourself for all the moments you diligently listened to this program.

Recall some of those affirmations now, the ones that mean the most to you, while I give you a moment of silence.

(Pause 30 seconds)

Then week 2 began and you got in touch with your hunger dial. You began acknowledging those times when you weren't really hungry at all and made notes about what you actually needed and maybe by now you've started fulfilling your needs in another way. What are some of those ways?

Then during the 3rd week, you got in touch with your feelings about your weight and how it's been for you so you could let go of those, and work with that same technique to bring into your life those behaviors that you do want.

We got right down to the heart of what's been causing your issue, during week four and everything became clear and you created new understandings within those moments, which transformed your experience.

During week 5, we started to work with the specific habits you want to bring into your life, and you recognize the value of drinking lots of water and water became a bigger part of your life. As did exercising during the sixth week.

After getting through this week, you realized you were halfway through the program, and it was a wonderful feeling to notice changes already starting to occur in your thinking and maybe even your body.

The following week, you added a healthy eating regimen to all the other habits that have been firmly in place for some time, and you feel a new sense of freedom to enjoy eating healthy from now on.

After creating these new habits, you learned a tool for being able to raise your metabolism and energize your body and deep breathing became a way of life for you.

During the 9th week, you knew you would definitely finish this program and it was becoming easier and easier to follow. You learned quite possibly one of the most life changing techniques ever created. This is when things really began to pick up. You wondered why this wasn't introduced in the first session, but later realized you wouldn't have the foundation or the wisdom of everything else you had learned.

You now enjoy using the swish routine every time you recognize limiting thoughts or behaviors and you feel inspired and motivated by the changes you have created. You are so glad you are finally changing your behaviors and seeing results, which you know are permanent.

Any of the extra fat or cellulite that decided it was going to hang around, had no choice but to vanish after week 10 when you diligently programmed your mind to remove it from your body.

Finally, you got to mold your body into the form and shape you have always wanted it to be. You have become better friends with your body than ever before. You realized how powerfully creative you are.

These changes you have made are permanent. They are who you are on every level and who you have always wanted to become. You are continuing to enjoy your new lifestyle of healthy eating, water drinking, and exercise.

You enjoy doing some form of deep breathing and relaxation for at least 15 minutes every day. You continue listening to your body and giving your body what it needs and giving yourself what you need.

You feel pride at knowing you have done something wonderful for yourself. Something that is life changing and will stick with you. Be sure to acknowledge any of the changes you've made in your life over the past several months. Any of the one's we've left out.

(Pause 30 seconds)

From this point forward, you'll enjoy listening to your hypnosis programs on a daily basis. You'll find that it supports you in achieving new levels of success all the time. Each and every day you're feeling healthier, you're feeling better about yourself, you're feeling better about your body and who you've become over the last 12 weeks.

Every day in every way you're getting better and better and it shows!

(Trance termination)

Download your scripts at www.VictoriaMGallagher.com/wlpbook

Forms

Client Agreement

Name: _____ Date: _____

Address: _____

City: _____ State: _____ Zip: _____

Home #: _____ Work #: _____ Cell #: _____

E-mail address: _____ Website: _____

Date of Birth: _____ Marital Status: _____

# of Children: _____ Occupation: _____

How did you hear about us? _____

_____

Referred by: _____

Reason for this session: _____

Other areas of interest: _____

Name of Physician: _____

Telephone #: _____

Hypnosis benefits are proven, and expectations are relative to client responsibility and commitment to succeed. Hypnosis is 80% effective in applications for behavior improvement and stress management necessary to good health and well-being. Hypnosis is a powerful tool in utilizing the resources of your mind and body to benefit you. Its benefits are relative to your participation, similar to that of a physician who prescribes medication / treatment, it works if you use it. In this regard, as a Hypnotherapist, 1) I do not diagnose, treat or cure disease, 2) I do not assess or evaluate Medical information, 3) I will determine if I am trained to work with your specific issues and, if not, I will refer you to other professionals, and 4) I am trained and certified in the skills of hypnosis and it's beneficial applications.

FORMS

Important! Hypnotherapist and client relationship responsibilities include the following statement of understanding. If I am presented with information that may be illegal or threat of harm to you or others, e.g. suicide, child abuse. I am legally obligated to report this possibility to Authorities.

I, _____

have reviewed the above stated information. I understand and accept the responsibilities of the Hypnotherapist/Client professional relationship that have been explained to me verbally and in written form

X _____

Download your forms at www.VictoriaMGallagher.com/wlpbook

Policies

FEES AND REFUND POLICY

Fees: One session; $_____. / _____-session-package; $_____ / _____ -session-package; $_____ / _____-session-package; $_____. Hypnosis is not guaranteed and there are no refunds. All policies apply in all cases. Appointments last _____. Time permitting, you may continue on longer at the rate of $_____ an hour.

SESSION CONTENT

Hypnosis is performed at the majority of sessions. However, it is not always necessary to perform hypnosis during every session. Sometimes we may need to work together in a totally conscious state of mind.

24-HOUR CANCELLATION POLICY

You will be required to pay for a "no show" or an appointment that is not cancelled within 24 hours.

15-MINUTE POLICY

If you are 15 minutes late it is considered a "no show." The 24-hour Cancellation Policy will apply. You will be charged for that session and we will reschedule your appointment.

RESCHEDULING

You may reschedule an appointment one time if you do it no less than 24-hours before your next appointment. You may only reschedule the same appointment one time. If you need to reschedule the rescheduled appointment, you will be required to pay for that appointment.

RESPONSIBLE CONVERSATIONS

Taking personal responsibility and being accountable for your life is the only path to true transformation. I will always ask you to speak from a place of responsibility, based on the choices you made leading up to the event you are faced with. An example would be being responsible for coming to your appointment on time. I understand you have "reasons" for things happening in your life. Please keep in mind you always have a choice. Even though you may get uncomfortable at times, I will ask you to face yourself truthfully.

SOLICITATION

Please refrain from any type of solicitation, enrollment, recruitment, or flirtation in my office. Any conversations that take the focus off of the services you are paying for taints the integrity of pureness of the therapy services you are paying for. If you have something you think I may be interested in, please put it in writing and if I am interested, I will contact you about it.

BARTER/TRADE

Should you have a service you feel is of value which you might like to trade for Hypnosis, that arrangement must be made with me well in advance of your session and is not to be discussed during your appointment.

DISTRACTIONS

In order for me to work with you effectively, you will need to come prepared to turn off cellular phones, hand-held devices, laptop computers, or other noisemakers. Please do not bring pets into my office (clients may have allergies.) Please make arrangements for childcare. You may bring a friend or spouse; however, it is advisable not to. You may bring water, but no food, cigarettes, drugs, or weapons.

I, _____
agree to adhere to all of the above policies.

X _____ Date _____

Download your forms at www.VictoriaMGallagher.com/wlpbook

S.M.A.R.T. Goal System Worksheet

STATED GOAL:

Is it SPECIFIC? How will you know that your goal has been completed?

_____

Is it MEASURABLE? How is it going to be measured?

What is point A? _____

What is point B? _____

Is it ACHIEVABLE? How do you know it is possible?

_____

_____

_____

Is it REALISTIC? How is this reachable given your timeline and resources?

_____

_____

_____

What is the TIMETABLE? Does my goal have a deadline? By when will I achieve it?

_____

Signed: _____ Date: _____

Download your forms at www.VictoriaMGallagher.com/wlpbook

Weight Loss Questionnaire

How long have you wanted to lose weight?
_____

At what age did you first notice weight gain?
_____

How much would you like to weigh?
_____

How many times do you eat per day?
_____

What time of day do you eat most?
_____

Does anyone in your household have a weight problem?
_____

What types of food normally do you have the most trouble with?
_____

How many times have you tried to lose weight in the past?
_____

For how long were your other attempts successful?
_____

Why did you regain the weight?
_____

What are the three main reasons for your wanting to lose weight?
_____
_____
_____

What is the one main reason you are currently overweight?
___

Would you be unable to lose weight at this time for any reason?
___

On what date would you like to achieve your goal?
___

Name other people who will appreciate or benefit from your new body.
___
___
___

List three fears you may have of continued weight gain.
___
___
___

What fear might you have of losing weight?
___
___
___

What forms of therapy have been tried before?
___

What worked?
___

What didn't work?
___

What is your opinion of previous therapies?
___

FORMS

Have you had any experience with hypnosis?
_____

What was it like?
_____

What is your work situation?
_____

Do you enjoy it?
_____

What are your sleeping, eating and exercise patterns?
_____

What situations or hobbies support you or help you relax?
_____
_____
_____

Download your forms at www.VictoriaMGallagher.com/wlpbook

Hand-outs

Week 1: Create an Affirmation Poster

What you'll need for homework are the following supplies: your notebook and pen, some inspiring music you like, colored pens or crayons, a piece of 8 1/2 by 11 or 11 by 14 white or light colored poster board, glue, a fitness magazine or two, and a pair of scissors.

After you have your list together, you'll then beautifully and creatively write them on your poster board with the colored pens and crayons. Cut a few images or words from your fitness magazine and paste them around your poster board. Get it just the way you like it.

Keep this poster board in the same location that you'll be doing your hypnosis every day. Someplace where you have easy access to it, and you can see it easily. Before beginning and after each day's hypnosis session, spend one minute looking at your poster board, the pictures, and the affirmations. If you feel drawn to do so, you may add new images or quotes or your own new affirmations to it along the way. You may feel like you need to change an affirmation, so it applies to you more. You may find an affirmation on one of the programs that you'll hear that you like and want to add it to your board. Just in case, when you make this board, be sure to leave room so you can add to it later.

Homework is an important part of the program. Do not underestimate the power of this simple tool. It works. Sometimes it's the simplest things in life that have the most power.

Download your worksheet at www.VictoriaMGallagher.com/wlpbook

Week 1: Weight Affirmations

I'm ready to be thin again.

It feels so good to have toned arms and legs.

I create an abundance of energy when I work out.

Exercise gives me a good feeling about myself.

I will soon see results and that motivates me to get up every morning.

My health is extremely important to me.

Taking care of my body gives me great confidence.

I am willing and committed to doing what it takes.

I deserve healthy food and a healthy body.

I will succeed at creating the body I've always wanted.

I can see myself fit into my smallest size clothes again.

It will feel so nice to show off my sexy body again.

My body is to be kept beautiful, healthy, and sexy.

I have fun and enjoy life when I am in good shape.

Water feels so refreshing and satisfying.

Water satisfies my food cravings.

I feel so good when I eat healthy.

I enjoy wearing skinny clothes that show off my incredible body.

Every time I exercise, I enjoy it more.

Every day I notice positive changes in my mind and my body.

I prefer to have a positive attitude.

It's time to be happy.

I am grateful for the ability to be active.

I nurture myself by living a healthy lifestyle.

My sleeping habits are improving.

Quality sleep is important to my overall health.

My body looks better when it's lean, firm, and strong.

As I strengthen my body, I strengthen my confidence and self-esteem.

Getting in shape makes life so much easier.

I can be an inspiration to others.

Getting in great shape is a worthy goal.

The success I achieve in my health will rub off on the rest of my life.

I am getting my whole life into balance.

I'm serious about my fitness routine and goals.

My body is my best friend.

Download your handout at www.VictoriaMGallagher.com/wlpbook

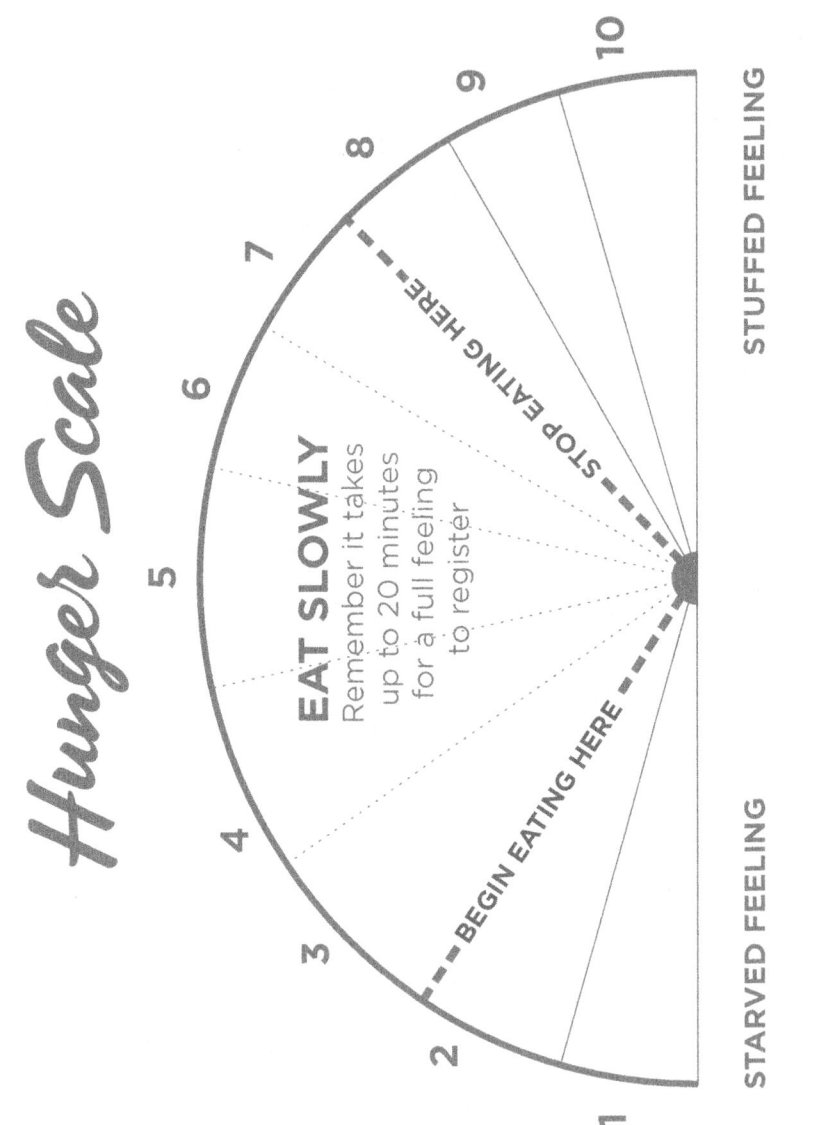

Hunger Scale

1 — STARVED FEELING
2 — BEGIN EATING HERE
3
4
5
6
7
8 — STOP EATING HERE
9
10 — STUFFED FEELING

EAT SLOWLY
Remember it takes up to 20 minutes for a full feeling to register

© 2019 Hyptalk.com, LLC

Download your handout at www.VictoriaMGallagher.com/wlpbook

Week 2: Emotional Eating Journal

To Bring Awareness to Unconscious Eating Behavior.

Keep this journal of every Time you Eat. Should Log Roughly 5x a Day for 7 Days.

Date	Time I Ate	How Hungry Am I When I Begin Eating? (1-10)	How Hungry Am I When I Stop Eating? (1-10)	What am I Feeling?	What Do I Want?	What Do I Need?

Download your worksheet at www.VictoriaMGallagher.com/wlpbook

Week 3: About Visualization

We all have 5 senses, hearing, sight, taste, touch, and smell. The 3 senses that we predominately use to represent things to ourselves are sight, hearing, and feeling.

The majority of people are predominantly visual, the next are predominantly auditory, they hear things, and the final group of people are more kinesthetic, feeling people.

All of these groups of people overlap in each of those areas. If you are not predominantly visual and you don't get pictures when you do this exercise, part of the reason may be because you hold a belief that you don't know how to visualize.

However, I'll bet that if I were to ask you to describe where you live or what color your car is or specific visual types of questions, your brain would present you with a quick picture in your mind before you answered my questions. At least this is usually the case. For example, what color is your car? If you said blue or red or whatever, how did you come up with your answer? How do you know it's blue? Are you remembering you bought a blue car and just hearing the word blue in your mind? Or does your mind quickly flash a picture of your car?

You may not be able to hold on to a picture in your mind or see it as close or sharp as you would like right now. However, this process that we are going to go through is great to remedy that situation. Yes, you can learn how to become more visually oriented. Additionally, you will be working with your other senses. When it comes to the swish part of the technique, maybe you will hear the changing of the frames or you will feel how they do it. You can do this. It just takes a little practice and you will get better at it and be able to create the things you want in your life.

Download your handout at www.VictoriaMGallagher.com/wlpbook

Week 5: Water

Recommended Reading: "Your Body's Many Cries For Water" by Fereydoon Batmanghelidj, M.D. which you will find on Amazon.com.

Humans may live for a month or more without food, but only a few days without water; only oxygen is more important. Each day, the body loses up to three quarts of water. A loss of only 10-20% of the body's water content could be fatal.

Fortunately, few of us are in danger of dehydration. However, there is much more to water than simply avoiding dehydration. Our bodies are designed to use pure water in every system to maintain life and health. Water is critical to everything we do. The body uses water for so many processes. Lack of water has been linked to all kinds of problems. Here are only a few of the processes the body utilizes water for:

- **Digestion:** Water is a component of gastric juices, pancreatic fluids, and saliva; Water transports nutrients through the digestive tract; and it dissolves nutrients.
- **Elimination:** Water dissolves waste products of cells, transports waste out of the body through kidneys, intestines, skin, and lungs.
- **Circulation:** Water transports nutrients and waste products in the blood and lymphatic fluids.
- **Temperature:** Water is a component of sweat to help the body maintain a constant temperature.
- **Absorption:** Water transports nutrients into the cells for utilization.
- **Lubrication:** Water lubricates the joints and your colon.

Lack of the proper amount of water can lead to problems with the functioning of these systems plus a whole lot more.

In our advanced society, we tend to think that we are getting our water intake by drinking any fluid that contains water, such as tea, coffee, alcohol, and other manufactured beverages.

While it is true that these beverages contain water, the other ingredients contained in these beverages, deprive the body of more water than is contained in the beverage, leaving you even more dehydrated. It is counterproductive to drink these beverages. If you do so, your body will require additional water to make up for the deprivation of water these beverages cause.

Let it be understood that by the time your mouth becomes dry, and you feel thirsty, you are already dehydrated. This is the final signal that the body urgently needs water. A good sign you are getting enough water is your urine has either little or no color to it. It has been said that many diseases have been caused by severe dehydration and they can be cured simply by drinking water. Obviously, this plays a major role on our stress because when our bodies are not physically functioning properly, stress is an inevitable response.

Download your handout at www.VictoriaMGallagher.com/wlpbook

HANDOUTS

Week 5: Water Drinking Weekly Journal

Monday ☐ ☐ ☐ ☐ ☐ ☐ ☐ ☐

Tuesday ☐ ☐ ☐ ☐ ☐ ☐ ☐ ☐

Wednesday ☐ ☐ ☐ ☐ ☐ ☐ ☐ ☐

Thursday ☐ ☐ ☐ ☐ ☐ ☐ ☐ ☐

Friday ☐ ☐ ☐ ☐ ☐ ☐ ☐ ☐

Saturday ☐ ☐ ☐ ☐ ☐ ☐ ☐ ☐

Sunday ☐ ☐ ☐ ☐ ☐ ☐ ☐ ☐

Download your worksheet at www.VictoriaMGallagher.com/wlpbook

Week 6: How to Get Back into the Exercise Habit

One of the biggest problems people face with their weight loss plans has to do with self-confidence. Self-confidence is knowing you have the ability to get things done.

Each time you say to yourself, "this week I am going to..." and you don't follow through on that, it reduces your self-confidence by a notch, making it that much harder to follow through the following week.

For example, if you are getting back into working out, let's say your ideal goal is to do cardio for 20 minutes three times a week and to work out with weights 40 minutes three times a week. However, let's say it's been more than 3 months since you have done any working out at all. The idea of this program might seem so overwhelming that you a) continue to put it off or b) get started on it for the standard two weeks and drop off. Does any of this sound familiar to you?

Of course, in either of those cases your self-confidence will go down and it becomes that much harder to get back into it again because you believe you will fail. One of the biggest motivating factors about anything you do in your life is having the belief in your ability to do it. Once you know you can and will do it, doing it is not as big of an issue. It's the doubt in whether you are ready to follow through or not that drags down your level of motivation. Right?

One of the things that I advise my clients to do is start with a 'ridiculously small' agreement to themselves that they know they can keep. Going back to the goal of working out, let's say the above example is where you would ideally like to be, but if you're not going to do it right now, what good is that? I am speaking directly to those who may have a hard time sticking to an exercise program consistently or getting one started. What I ask is this: "How much of that goal would you be willing to commit to this week? Minimum participation can be as little as 30 seconds a day." And usually what most will agree to at this point is anywhere between 5 minutes to 10 minutes a day.

Here is why I believe it would be better to do 30 seconds a day, than nothing at all:

- If you are starting from square one, where you haven't moved your body at all to moving your body vigorously for even as little as 30 seconds a day, there are a number of benefits you will get from starting out in this small way.
- First of all, the main point of this exercise is to build your self-confidence back up to the ultimate level where you know you will do whatever you say you are going to do. (I recommend keeping ALL of your agreements as well.) Even if it is a tiny little thing you have completed. Completing anything will enhance your self-confidence so that maybe the following week you will add more time to this goal.
- Secondly, you raise your metabolism by even a slight amount.
- Third, you will be putting exercise into your conscious awareness.
- Fourth, you will be creating a daily positive habit. Activity is a great affirmation to your body that you are doing something to take care of yourself and toward your goal.
- And finally, without you consciously trying to do anything at all, your body will tell you that it is ready for more. Even if these 30 seconds you spend seem difficult at first, you will increase your endurance by doing something consistently and will eventually need to do more to receive the same satisfaction.

Everything we have talked about so far deals with something you will do at a conscious level. What I highly recommend is to go into hypnosis for a minimum of 15 minutes on a consistent daily basis and work on your goal at a subconscious level. Let your subconscious mind do 90% of the work. I ask you to consciously participate with the 10% you do have control over. As you continue listening to your goal and visualize and even feel yourself exercising and being in the best shape of your life, these thoughts will eventually take over and become your new behaviors.

When you are working at a subconscious level, I further recommend you listen to your hypnosis program at a time just before you work out because it will help increase your motivation. I don't like to dictate when you "should" do something or what is right or wrong or bad or good. These are recommendations and what I have seen work for others. If something else works better for you, go for it.

I do suggest however, there are benefits to working out and doing hypnosis in the morning (or whenever you wake up) that are not available to you at the end of the day. One is that working out on an empty stomach causes you to burn fat first, rather than the protein and carbohydrates you have been eating all day. Secondly, working out in the morning will give you more energy throughout the day. You turn up your metabolism when you are active, which helps you to capitalize on any potential fat burning activity you do that day, as opposed to right before you fall asleep when the smallest number of calories are burned.

Some of the benefits of doing hypnosis in the morning are that you are less likely to fall asleep again after you have been asleep all night. You are already somewhat in a hypnotic state when you first wake up and therefore you can take advantage of that state you are already in to listen to your hypnosis program.

To recap, I recommend starting a ridiculously small workout program to build up a habit and a sense of self-confidence. Let your powerful subconscious mind do most of the work by feeding it the suggestions that will support your overall workout goal.

My final recommendation is to reward yourself with something positive. Choose a reward that is in line with your overall health goal, not food. Food has been used since the beginning of time as a celebration activity and so it is ingrained in our minds to celebrate our successes with food. However, all that does is reinforce your old beliefs and your old behaviors about food.

Here are a few suggestions to reward yourself: Take a drive to a nearby beautiful place in nature. Buy yourself a new outfit. Buy yourself a book you've wanted to read. Buy yourself a new music Mp3, or even some more hypnosis Mp3s that will help you continue to feel good about yourself.

Download your handout at www.VictoriaMGallagher.com/wlpbook

HANDOUTS

Week 6: Simple Exercise Journal

To Bring Awareness to Unconscious Eating Behavior.
Keep this journal of every Time you Eat. Should Log Roughly 5x a Day for 7 Days.

Date/Date	Time of Day	Activity	Length of Time	How Did I Feel?
Sunday _____				
Monday _____				
Tuesday _____				
Wednesday _____				
Thursday _____				
Friday _____				
Saturday _____				

Download your worksheet at www.VictoriaMGallagher.com/wlpbook

Week 7: Nutrition

Eating right, especially during stressful times is not only important in regard to getting the proper nutrition for vitamins and minerals sake. It is extremely important to your digestive system. When the stress response is activated, blood is drawn away from the digestive system. The flow of digestive juices is halted. Thus, digestion and absorption processes are altered. If you react to stress by overeating, particularly an overindulgence in fatty foods, you are putting stress on your digestive system. A few guidelines to keep in mind to eliminate stress to your digestive system are:

- Eat a number of small meals rather than fewer larger meals. Besides aiding your digestion, this will keep your blood-sugar level up, which will help you to avoid getting fatigued.
- Gradually include more and more fiber to your diet. Your system will need about 2 - 3 weeks to adjust to the change.
- Eat breakfast. Studies show that people who skip breakfast tend to overeat the rest of the day.
- During a stressful time, don't forget to eat. This can lead to starving all day and overeating at night.

Following these guidelines and developing sound nutritional habits will increase your resistance to stress. The key word is habit. Don't start some kind of diet program you do not feel you could do for your whole life. Diets are temporary and most people end up in a worse condition after dieting than had they simply continued their normal eating habits. Changing how you eat permanently, is what works permanently. It is as simple as that.

Some of us cope with stress by eating food; sometimes lots of food. Others cannot eat anything as the first signs of stress appear. Some of us cope with stress by eating ice cream or potato chips. Others cope by eating carrot sticks or an apple.

Proper nutrition is one of the first things that gets tossed aside under stress.

You may feel like you are too busy because you are on the go all the time, so you turn to fast food. Or you may start snacking on garbage. Even worse, skip meals all together.

Unfortunately, by eating poorly you're making a bad situation worse.

A diet consisting of the same foods every day or eating less than 1000 calories a day or consisting mainly of high fat and high sugar will eventually result in nutritional deficiencies that may cause illness.

There are some foods which activate the stress response in you. Foods that contain caffeine and foods with sugar.

Not only do people deprive themselves of normal amounts of nutrition while under stress, but the body needs some nutrients in great amounts when under stress

Especially during stressful times, high levels of certain vitamins are needed to maintain proper functioning of the nervous and endocrine systems. These vitamins are vitamin C and the vitamins found in the B-Complex vitamin. Deficiencies of vitamins B-1, B-5, and B-6 can lead to anxiety, depression, insomnia, and cardiovascular weaknesses, while B-2 and niacin deficiencies have been known to cause stomach irritability and muscular weakness. Their depletion lowers your tolerance to and ability to cope with stress.

The need for vitamin C increases when under stress. Vitamin C is stored in the adrenal gland. After the gland releases adrenal hormones as part of the stress response, the supply needs to be replenished. The production of adrenal hormones is accelerated by vitamin C. Vitamin C is needed for the synthesis of the thyroid hormone. Thyroid hormone production regulates the body's metabolism. Thus, when the metabolic rate increases under stress, so does the need for vitamin C.

The point of eating a balanced meal is to get all the vitamins your body needs on a daily basis to function properly. Knowing and being aware of which foods contain these vitamins and what the vitamins do, may motivate you to eat the foods that provide you what your body needs. The B vitamins are supplied in protein rich foods, such as meats and cheeses. Vitamin C is found in citrus fruits, broccoli, strawberries, tomatoes, cauliflower, and green peppers.

Download your handout at www.VictoriaMGallagher.com/wlpbook

Week 7: Healthy Eating Plan

	Breakfast	Lunch	Dinner	Snacks
Monday				
Tuesday				
Wednesday				
Thursday				
Friday				
Saturday				
Sunday				

Download your worksheet at www.VictoriaMGallagher.com/wlpbook

Induction Scripts

Walking Through a Desert

Imagine yourself walking through a desert. You are walking barefoot on the sand, which is so fine and warm. You feel the warmth of the sand as it envelops your every step and oozes between each of your toes. As you continue your journey through the desert, you feel a slight warm breeze. You feel the tiny sand granules brushing up against your shins and your calves causing a slight tingling sensation. Looking out into the horizon, you see the desert appears as though it continues on for an eternity. Off in the distance you see the sun. It is a bright orangish-yellow. It gives off a golden glow all around it and extends into a purple haze throughout the entire sky.

As the sun is beginning to set, it seems to melt into the desert floor. If you look off to your right, you see a moon beginning to appear. You stop walking for a moment and take a closer look at this moon. A large moon that has a bluish tint and a glow of a white ring all around it.

You've never seen the moon looking quite as beautiful and magnificent as it does in this moment, you are simply mesmerized and becoming relaxed simply by letting your eyes bring the moon into full view. Allow your eyes to bring this moon closer and closer into focus. Even closer now. So close ... you feel as though you can reach right out and touch the moon. The moon is right next to you.

You feel a sensation of coolness coming over you. The white ring around the moon is clearly a white energy field of light and this white light extends out into where you are standing and completely outlines your entire body. You feel an electrical tingling feeling running up and down throughout your entire body. It feels as though you have joined the same energy force as the moon, and it is pulling you closer and closer toward it. It feels safe and you have no fear about walking even closer toward the moon and putting your hand out to touch it. Go ahead and put your hand out and touch the surface of the moon. It feels cool and kind of chalky...kind of pasty... In a moment I'm going to ask you to take a step forward and when you do, you'll be stepping onto the moon. Notice it has a relaxing affect upon you.

Go ahead and take that step now. Ahh, how relaxing. The moon begins to float upward. You have no care in the world about this. You feel completely relaxed and at ease. You are floating through the sky. You see the stars as it is nighttime and dark. The stars shine so brightly. As you float higher and higher, you notice the stars are becoming closer and closer. As they get closer, they become clearer and brighter than you've ever seen them before. The brighter they become, the more deeply relaxed you become. Listen to the silence. There is complete silence where you are. It is so quiet. It is so quiet ... you can even hear the chatter inside your own mind.

As the stars become brighter, your inner voices in your own mind get more and more quiet. It's quite amazing to notice how much noise is usually happening within your own mind until you tune in and listen to it. You see the stars so close as you pass them by, you can only see one or two at a time as you realize that they are actually other planets with the most amazing coloring.

Bright blues, greens, yellows, and purples are swirled together in all different styles and shapes. The moon that is floating further up into the universe is beginning to slow down, slowing way down. As it does, you notice, even this far out into the universe there are big white fluffy clouds all around you and you can use the clouds to transport you to the other planets all around you.

You pull yourself on to one of the clouds and allow yourself to drift for a while through outer space while you find yourself a new planet to visit. It's so hard to choose. They are all so intriguing. As a matter of fact, they are not only bright and beautiful, but now you are even able to notice they each have their own wonderful scent. One of them smells like a rose. Allow yourself to breathe in the beautiful aroma of roses. Another one smells like fresh pine trees.

You stop here and explore and so you step down off of the cloud and step onto this planet. The feeling under your feet is a squishy, soft, rubbery-like feeling. Your feet sink into the surface and leave an imprint with each step you take, and you begin your journey to explore this planet. Up ahead in the distance you notice it gets darker and darker almost like the planet just fades into complete nothingness. You feel intrigued by what is ahead of you so much ... you begin to walk closer toward the darkness.

You feel completely safe and secure. For you know that in this place, there is nothing that can bother you or harm you in any way. You have everything you need to feel powerful. You have everything you need to feel safe. You have everything you need to feel happy. You have everything you need to allow yourself to enjoy every aspect of your journey without any worries at all.

You continue walking toward this area that is dark and empty and find yourself walking into total nothingness. You find yourself with nothing under your feet. You look all around you and notice the planets have disappeared, the moon, the clouds, the bright colors, have all disappeared. It is quiet.

You find yourself slowly sinking...going down...sinking deeper. There is nothing around you at all. You feel completely safe and peaceful. The only thing that is happening since there is nothing else is you are going down, deeper and deeper. It's a pleasant feeling. Very relaxing. A light feeling of euphoria envelops you and you are feeling so good. You allow yourself to float and drift down in a peaceful way. You no longer feel like you are in your body. Since you do not see a thing, you haven't been able to see your body for many miles. Since you are so relaxed and drifting down in such a pleasant peaceful way, you haven't been able to feel your body and so it feels as though you left it somewhere and you are left with only one thing. You are left with your higher self. The part of you that can and will do anything you desire. It is the part of you which follows directions.

If you desire to do so, you may go ahead and give a command to this part of yourself. You may ask it to do anything you desire it to do for you and it will listen and it will grant you whatever you ask it to do if it is for your highest good and the highest good of everyone else. Go ahead, do this now... Wonderful...

Something else your higher self can assist you with is, it can provide you with answers to any questions you may have. For this higher self has access to an all-knowing entity called universal intelligence. To get the answer to any question you may have, all you have to do is ask the question and then be silent and wait for the answer. You need do nothing else. Ask a question and wait. Let's go ahead and do this now. Ask a question and when you have finished just be quiet. Great.

Download your scripts at www.VictoriaMGallagher.com/wlpbook

Down the Stairs

Close your eyes...Relax...and let your imagination guide you for the next little while into a special place where all of your desires become a reality...all of them. Places where magnificent changes take place...if...you are willing and open and allow it to happen.

Let your mind sink now and experience this place in your mind where all of your dreams can be completely fulfilled...if...you are ready. Are you ready? If you are ready then say "yes" and let that word, "yes" echo throughout your mind.

Hear my words with your own voice, echoing over and over and over again. Say "yes" again and from this point forward, every time you close your eyes and hear the word "yes" with either your own voice or mine... that word, "yes" puts you deeper into trance. That's right. You affirm and re-affirm any and all of the suggestions I'm about to give you by repeating that word, "yes" in your mind.

"Yes" means you are willing and open to having the changes take place in your life that I'm going to talk about in a few moments. Are you willing and open? Do you trust your mind is powerful enough to create the changes you want to make? Say "yes." Good. Go deeper and deeper and deeper and deeper. Yes...Yes...Yes.

You are relaxed. In a moment, I'm going to take you 10x deeper than you are right now. Are you ready to go 10x deeper? Good... begin by imagining yourself at the top of a beautiful staircase. Before moving a muscle, notice your breathing for a moment. Notice your breathing. How does it feel? Does it feel soft and easy? Each breath is sending a warm and relaxing vibration throughout your body.

How does your body feel? Are there any areas in your body that need a little extra relaxation? Go ahead and breathe in gently and as you breathe out imagine you are sending that out breath down to wherever it is in your body that needs that

INDUCTION SCRIPTS

extra relaxation. Spend a little more time concentrating on your breathing.

Breathe gently and slowly. This breathing is the direct route to your total relaxation. Good... notice your body and the way it feels. Can you feel a little tingling sensation anywhere in your body? Or numbness? This is a great way to tell whether your body is becoming relaxed or not.

In any case, you are doing fine and we were just about to take a nice slow stroll down a set of stairs so when I tell you to, you'll take your first step to stair #10 of this set of 10 stairs and each time you take a step down to a new stair you will feel the step sending a wave of relaxation throughout your body and you will go twice as relaxed as you were before. Twice as deep on every step until you reach the bottom of the stairway which is filled with soft fluffy clouds that will gently hold your body safely and comfortably and allow you to float in this state of trance.

Let's begin ...

10 ... Step down and feel yourself go deeper ... good ... 9 ... and deeper still ... double your relaxation ... 9 ... very nice ...8 ... feel the wave of relaxation moving through you ... 7 ... you're doing great ... and deeper still ... 6 ... feeling so good ... feeling that wave of relaxing energy moving through each cell of your body ... 5 ... that's right ... feel yourself going down ... down ... down ... 4 ... and deeper and deeper and deeper ... 3 ... you are so comfortably relaxed ... you feel you may float away ... 2 ... never felt quite this peaceful before and feeling better all the time ... and now ready for the ultimate feeling of beautiful restful hypnotic rest ... get ready to take that last step ... 1 ... good ...

Lie back on the clouds ... and allow them to take you wherever they may go ... while your subconscious mind is perfectly open and receptive to hearing and receiving the suggestions to make the changes you want to make in your life.

Healing Light

Close your eyes and relax. Uncross your arms and legs. Lay back on the floor or sit upright in a chair. Take some deep breaths. Breathe in slowly through your nose and exhale through your mouth. Let your mind be calm and peaceful. Breathe. Let the sound of my voice be all you are aware of.

Allow a ball of light...any color you choose...to enter your mind. Allow the light to enter your body through the top of your head. As it flows through your head, feel the warmth of the energy as it relaxes your mind. As the healing force travels inside your head, it relieves any anxiety you may have. Any thoughts about your day melt away. Any guilt about the day just passed simply disappears. Any fears about what the future will bring effortlessly fades away.

You are right here, right now, and you are safe.

Breathe.

Allow this healing light to relax your forehead...your eyebrows... your eyelids...Allow your cheekbones to relax...and your nose... and your mouth...your jaws...your lips. Breathe. The light travels down your neck, relaxing the back of your neck...the front of your neck...and your throat. You feel the warmth of the energy sending a tingling renewing sensation throughout your neck.

Let this ball of light branch off into your shoulders, relaxing them completely. Breathe. Let it go down your arms...your upper arms...your elbows...your forearms...relaxing....and the palms of your hands. Allow the warm tingling sensation to spread across your palms and into your fingers. Feel the vibration of your body as it relaxes more and more deeply. Breathe.

The ball of light now goes into your chest area and relaxes any tension there and into your heart, cleansing it to make room for more love. Feel the warmth of the energy as it moves through your spinal column relaxing every vertebra...slowly...one by one...

The healing ball of light moves into your stomach, easing any tension there and relaxing it completely. It enters your buttocks.

You feel the tension releasing. Relax...let go and breathe. The light branches off into your thighs, relaxing. It then travels through to your knees...your calves...your ankles...relaxing.

Finally, the ball of light has reached your feet. Feel the healing light sending a warm energy throughout every cell of your feet and toes. Visualize yourself as completely cleansed and this light now leaves your body going back down into the earth leaving through your toes...You are completely relaxed...warm... safe...and comfortable.

Download your scripts at www.VictoriaMGallagher.com/wlpbook

Healthy Body

Prepare to enter a deep state of relaxation. Begin by adjusting your body into a comfortable position. Lay down. Stretch out your legs and place your arms out at your sides away from your body with your palms up. Gently close your eyes. Take in a slow soft deep breath. Exhale slowly. Breathe in again. This time hold your breath for a moment until you hear me say release it. When you let the breath out this time, imagine that any negative thoughts feelings or energies are coming out of your body. Do that now... release it... good. Breathe in an even deeper breath and hold it again until I say release it.

Imagine you're breathing in calming relaxing energy. Letting out stress and tension and release it. Good. One last time on your own. That's good. Your breathing is relaxing you. For the remainder of this session, every breath you take from now on will continue to relax you deeper and deeper. Take one more breath with me. Cause your body to feel more relaxed than before you took that breath. Breathe in and relax deeper and let it out. You are even more deeply relaxed than before.

You have conditioned your mind to be able to relax on command simply by breathing in and setting your intention on relaxation. You're creating a healthy environment within and all around your lungs as you continue focusing on breathing in this natural healthy way you're doing right now.

Let's take this relaxation you're experiencing a little deeper, focus all of your attention on your heartbeat. Tune in and notice the rhythm of your heartbeat. Put a picture of your heart in your mind's eye. See it beating in a normal healthy way. Notice how stable your heart rate is. When you relax this way and breathe deeply on a regular basis you restore all the cells in your body to their natural healthy state. The flow of the oxygen now present in your body, causes you to release stress. You're becoming calm and more peaceful. You take control of your life right now and all of the changes you want to make by simply relaxing and getting in touch with that part of your mind that creates whatever you desire. You're making time for this each and every day. You enjoy this time. You enjoy taking care of yourself on every level; mentally, emotionally, physically, and spiritually.

Continue to focus on your breathing now and throughout your day. Let's take this relaxation a little deeper now by focusing all of your attention on your eyes. Focus intently now on your eyelids and you're going to cause your eyelids to become relaxed so that when I tell you to and not until then you will try to open your eyes and find you cannot.

First, we're going to get them relaxed. Loose and limp. Loose and limp. So relaxed that you will not be able to open your eyes. Your eyelids are becoming stuck together. Your eyelids are beginning to feel like one piece of skin. Your eyes will not open even if you tried. Want that to happen. Make that happen.

In a moment, you'll get to find out just how powerful your mind really is. You will try to open your eyes and find that you cannot. While keeping in mind you know you could open your eyes if you wanted to. Right now, they're feeling too tired too relaxed that they want to stay closed. Now try to open your eyes and find that you cannot. Try a little harder. Stop trying and relax. Relax your eyes. Go deeper. Deeper relaxed.

To go even deeper relaxed, I'm going to suggest that you open and close your eyes several more times. Every time you open your eyes and then close them again, you will double your relaxation.

Now, open your eyes. Close your eyes and go deeper, even deeper. Again, open your eyes and close them again. Double your relaxation. Double your relaxation... Go even deeper. Again, open your eyes and close them. Go deep. Let your body completely let go and relax.

Every muscle in your body is completely loose and limp and this feels good. Your mind is powerful when you achieve this level of relaxation. You allow yourself to remain at this deep level of relaxation simply by focusing on the sound of my voice and the background music. While you may be able to detect some other sounds, any sounds that might ordinarily disturb you will only have a relaxing effect on you.

Any time you notice any sounds around you they only cause you to go deeper relaxed. At the same time, my voice will influence your subconscious mind in a wonderful way. My voice will travel into the deepest levels of your subconscious mind to create the changes you desire to make in your life. My voice will always stimulate a relaxing soothing calming feeling within you. So that you will immediately begin to associate my voice with relaxation the moment you begin to listen. You will notice yourself being able to achieve deeper levels of relaxation each time you practice.

(Optional imagery)

Allow your mind to take you to a beautiful place. A place you choose that is safe and warm and comfortable. A place out in nature... A place that creates and even deeper sense of calm and peace within you... Take a moment to create this special place.

Now that you've created this special place, imagine you are lying down on the ground. Notice your level of connection with this place. You now deepen your level of connection simply by taking a couple of slow deep breaths. Notice the way that the ground beneath you energizes your body. What an incredible feeling to feel the very life force energy of the universe flowing inside of you. Restoring your body to perfect health.

As you breathe in image you are breathing in the atmosphere around you. Every breath you take causes the colors you see around you to become more and more vivid, bright, and beautiful. As you look out into the distant sky, you will notice a rainbow. You allow each color of the rainbow to blend together and form one column of white light that reaches down from the sky and touches the top of your head. Feel the way this light feels.

As it pours into the top of your head, relaxing, healing light. Cleansing every cell in your body as it continues to flow down from the top of your head and into your forehead. Smoothing out the little space between your eyebrows. Spreading out through your entire face, your nose, your cheeks, your chin, and your jaws. Relaxing every muscle and nerve. Feel this light moving down your neck. The back of your neck... The front of your neck... Absorbing any tension and tightness.

Feel this light moving down into your shoulders, relaxing your shoulders. Let your shoulders become loose and limp. Feel this relaxing energy traveling through each of your arms, your hands, and down to the tips of your fingers. From your neck and shoulders down into the upper part of your back. Traveling down and around each vertebra and into your lower back. From your neck and shoulders down into your chest and your abdomen and your stomach. Relax your stomach muscles. Relax your stomach muscle completely.

Feel this wave of energy extending into your buttock muscles. Releasing and relaxing that area completely... Your thighs feel this energy. The muscles within your thighs are relaxing. Your knees, your calves and into your heels... Feel all this energy concentrated into that one central location, your heels. Move all that energy into the arches of your feet. Feel it in the balls of your feet. Your toes... You have utilized this healing light to relax you completely. Now send it out from your toes back down into the ground as you remember where you lay out in nature.

Download your scripts at www.VictoriaMGallagher.com/wlpbook

My Elman

All right. So, let yourself relax into a comfortable position... with your arms open and out at your sides... your legs uncrossed with your feet about 6 inches or so apart. Take in a deep breath in through your nose... Let it out slowly.... as you exhale ... allow your eyes to close... Allow your entire body to relax... Let your entire body relax... from your head to your toes... As you do so... close your eyes tighter and tighter... that's right....

As you feel your entire body relaxing from your head to your toes ... close your eyes tighter and tighter.... as you close your eyes tighter and tighter your body relaxes more and more... more and more. as you relax more and more your eyes close tighter and tighter.... You don't have to close them quite so tight... as all the muscles of your eyes relax more and more your body relaxes more and more...

The muscles of your eyes are so relaxed... so relaxed that you can't be bothered to use them.... Don't use them... let them relax more and more... more and more so that you can't be bothered to use them.... Relax and let go... so that you can't be bothered to use your eyes at all.... Don't use them at all....

In a moment, I'm going to ask you to try to open your eyes and when I do so, you will simply try to open them you won't really open them you'll allow yourself to experience a feeling like you can't open your eyes. Each time we do this, you'll find yourself believing more and more strongly that you can't open your eyes even though you know you could open them if you wanted to.

This exercise will cause you to relax into a profound deep state of relaxation. Ready, let's try it once. Go ahead now and try them... remember like we said, try them, but only so much that they may only barely come open. Ready? Once again, try to open your eyes... Stop trying and relax. You are doing well...

Now I'm going to count from one to three and this time your eyes will open on the count of three and then I'll count back from three to one and they'll close again, and you'll double

INDUCTION SCRIPTS

that feeling of relaxation. One, two, three... eyes open... and three, two, one... eyes closed... and deeper relaxed, doubling the feeling of relaxation... deeply relaxed... going even deeper... Relax.

Any time you hear me say the word relax, you will relax more deeply than before. Relax. Relax. Relax. In a moment we'll be opening and closing the eyelids again ... each time you do, you'll notice yourself dropping into an even deeper state of relaxation.... Relax. Completely. Relax ... all the way around your eyes... your eyelids, your eyeballs... and every single muscle that controls the movement of your eyes....

I'm going to count from one to three and your eyes will open and from three to one and your eyes will close and you'll go even deeper relaxed, one two three, eyes open... and three, two, one, eyes closed... and deeper relaxed, doubling the feeling of relaxation. Deep, deep, deep... going even deeper now...

Let go of any remaining tension... completely relax... relax more and more...relax your eyes more and more. So much so that the muscles will not want to work. Let them relax, more and more... more and more, so that you put them out of action temporarily. They won't work. They just won't want to. Try to open your eyes... and even if you opened your eyes and are closing them again now ... notice how you have doubled that feeling of relaxation. Very relaxed all the way around your eyes.

I will now begin to count from one to three and they will open and from three to one and they will close again, and you will double that feeling of relaxation again. One, two, three, eyes open... and three, two, one, eyes closed and deeply relaxed. Deep, deep, deeper relaxed.... Doubling that feeling of relaxation. Your entire body relaxes. All your facial muscles... your chin and your jaw muscles. Down through the muscles of your neck. To your shoulders and your shoulder joints. Your shoulder blades. Every bone and joint in your spine. Every muscle and nerve in your back. That's right. Going even deeper. Deep, deep, deeply relaxed. From your shoulders, down each arm and hand, down to your fingertips and from your shoulders through your chest and stomach muscles and down to the tips of your toes, completely relaxed.

Now ... see the number 100 in your imagination. See that number 100 out in front of you. In a moment I'm going to count backwards from 100 and you'll simply repeat the numbers right along with me out loud. With each number that we count, your feelings of relaxation will double deeper and deeper into relaxation. That's right. As you're counting and hearing your own voice, hearing the sound of your own voice will bring you into an even deeper state of relaxation. Once again, see that number 100 out in front of you in your imagination Ready? 100 (then you say 100 right along with me.)

I'll be saying a few words between numbers to help you deepen your relaxation and you'll drift off into a deep state of hypnotic rest. 99 ... deeper and deeper.... 98 doubling the feeling of relaxation... going deeper...97 ... even deeper... doubling the feelings of relaxation. Go deep. 96 ... even deeper now... let go.

Let those numbers fade away. Deeper and deeper. Allow those numbers to fade away. Deep, deep, deep. Let those numbers fade away. Deeper and deeper. Good. You're now in a sleep like state, where your subconscious mind is open and receptive to all of the suggestions, I'm about to give you. Let yourself relax and float and drift in this wonderful hypnotic state.

Download your scripts at www.VictoriaMGallagher.com/wlpbook

INDUCTION SCRIPTS

Progressive Muscle Relaxation

In a moment ... you'll be relaxing every muscle in your body... which will cause you to feel a beautiful sense of calm and peace ... in your body ... your mind ... your emotions ... and your soul ... a wonderful feeling you'll be able to bring forth whenever you think about it ... from this point forward ... many people spend their whole lives in search of this kind of peace of mind ... which you'll be creating for yourself in the next little while ... and even you may have never experienced such a depth of relaxation as you are about to experience ... give yourself this time ... to experience yourself ... to experience lightness ... weightlessness ... pleasure. It's so important that you take time to do this...

Each day you allow yourself this opportunity ... to go within ... you achieve deeper states than ever before ... and you will be able to access a state of trance more quickly and easily ... let's begin ...

By now you will have adjusted your body into a comfortable quiet place where you will remain undisturbed for the next 25 minutes. You can sit in a chair with your back straight and your feet firmly planted in front of you or lie down, whichever works better for you and is more comfortable ... so long as you will remain slightly awake throughout this entire process ...

Keep your arms and legs uncrossed in an open body position ... Tune into your breathing ... place one hand on your lower abdomen ... when you breathe, make sure your breath is filling up your entire abdomen and you are breathing slowly ... Inhale to a slow count of four ... then holding that breath ... and exhaling to a slow count of eight ... take a moment to pay attention to your breathing ... and imagine you are breathing in relaxation and breathing out any tension or stress ... I'll be silent for one minute to give you some time to practice breathing in such a way that your abdomen is rising and falling with each breath ...

(Pause one minute)

Breathe naturally. Notice your level of relaxation, which is getting deeper and deeper all the time.

Direct your attention to the top of your head... to your scalp ... to the skin that covers your scalp ... feel this area and notice any of the sensations in this area around the top of your head. You may notice your pulsation at the top of your head, or you may notice a tingling sensation.

Do whatever you need to do to cause this part of your body, the top of your head to become calm and relaxed. Focus on your forehead. Cause your forehead to become tense by raising your eyebrows and hold that position for the next 5 seconds... and now relax your forehead... feel your forehead smoothing out and becoming limp and relaxed.

Place your attention on your eyes and close your eyes tightly. Hold for a count of 5. Relax your eyes. Let go of all the tiny little muscles that surround your eyes. Allow this part of your body to relax deeper. Direct all your attention now to your jaw muscles. Cause this part of your body to become tense by clinching your teeth together, holding for a few seconds... and relax your jaw completely... you allow your jaw to become even more relaxed by allowing your lips and your teeth to part slightly.

Allow your jaw to go limp and droop down and relax. This is a wonderful signal to help the rest of your body begin to relax as well. Moving down your body let yourself feel any tension in the back of your neck by slowing bending your neck back and hold that tension for 5 seconds. Release the tension in your neck by taking in a deep breath now, letting your neck fall naturally into a comfortable position and expel all the air from your lungs, breathing out any remaining feelings of tightness. Relax your neck.

Direct your attention to your shoulders, another area where you might store a lot of your tension, so let's feel that tension by bringing your shoulders upward toward your ears and hold. Breathe in again and let your shoulders drop down to a position that feels perfect and as you breathe out become even more relaxed as your shoulders rest comfortably in their relaxed position.

INDUCTION SCRIPTS

When your body relaxes this way, your mind and your emotions follow along and become just as relaxed while you focus all of your attention on relaxing each of these muscles in your body. You will now focus your attention on your arms. Feel the muscles in your upper arms and your lower arms. Tense these muscles by stretching your arms downward, alongside your legs, stiffening and tensing the muscles within your arms and hold. Release your arms, let them go loose and limp. Imagine all the energy drain out of your arms, so you feel you couldn't lift them even if you tried.

We now come to your hands. Cause your hands to become tense by making a fist. Hold that fist tight for a moment... and release it. Feel the warmth and relaxation spreading throughout your hands and your fingers. You might even feel a slight tingling sensation.

Then, turn your attention toward the muscles in your back area. Cause these muscles in your back to become tense by pushing your shoulders back a little and feel that tension for about 5 seconds. Release it. Let go of your back and allow relaxation to move throughout that entire area.

Focus on your chest by taking in and holding a deep breath. Breathe in and hold your breath to a count of five and when you let the breath out, let your lungs and your chest feel the relief of relaxation. Breathe naturally, allowing each breath you take from now on to cause you to drift into a deeper state of relaxation. What a beautiful, healthy state of calm, which is becoming deeper all the time.

Move on down to your abdomen and squeeze the muscles of your abdomen, suck in those muscles, feel them tight and tense... and hold... and now release them. Feel them more and relaxed. Feel your breath sending waves of relaxation into your belly. Feel it and go even deeper. Next, tense the muscles of your buttocks. Squeeze your buttocks muscles and hold. Let them go. Relax your buttocks muscles.

Now direct your focused attention to your thighs. Tighten these muscles in your thighs for a few seconds. Release your thighs completely. Let them go completely loose and limp. Feeling good, feeling relaxed.

Coming to your calves ... tense these muscles and hold the tension... and release the tension... feel the waves of comfort and relaxation which has spread throughout your entire body. You now go into an even deeper state of relaxation by paying close attention to your feet. Feel your feet and point your toes as if you were squeezing out that last little bit of tension ... hold it for a moment...

As you let your feet go and let them relax completely, imagine yourself as pure energy. That can look like anything you like. This energy which has been inside of this body. You can float up now, right out of your body. You let your body go and rest peacefully, while you, the real you, the purest essential part of your being, which you may call your spirit, or whatever feels best for you, this part of you can now float and let your body be peaceful. Float up and leave your body so it can receive the most benefit from this relaxation. Your mind and your emotions are leaving your body, so your body can rejuvenate itself.

Imagine yourself in any way you wish, that you are energy, your spiritual self, looking down at your body which is sitting or lying so peacefully. You're up there above your body about six feet or so above. You now draw a brilliant illuminating white protective light all around your body. You may want to add some color to this white light like purple flecks or gold sparkle.

While you see yourself with this glowing beautiful light all around you, you feel much more peaceful and relaxed. You will remain in this dreamy drowsy state for as long as you like or until the time when I ask you to bring your attention back to waking consciousness. At the time I ask you to come back to full waking consciousness, you will become aware of your body again and everything will return back to normal.

For now, you'll continue to let everything in this physical realm go completely. As a matter of fact, you can use my voice to bring you deeper and deeper into relaxation. You allow my voice to affect and become your own internal voice. The words I say to you from now on will have a profound effect on you.

INDUCTION SCRIPTS

My words strongly influence your thoughts, your behaviors, your feelings, and help you make changes in your life that you desire. The more you listen, the more influence my voice will have upon you and the deeper you will go into hypnosis. Your subconscious mind hears my words and these words become your predominant thoughts.

Any of your old thoughts, which promote negative behaviors, lose any of the power you once gave them. You may hear a negative thought, and you are now able to turn down the volume on that thought and turn up the volume on the thoughts that support you in creating what you desire.

This state of relaxation you are in, is the most powerful state you can experience. You were born with the most amazing tool ever known to man, your subconscious mind, where you can create anything you want. It's always nice to have someone guide you into this state.

Know that you have created this simply by listening and following the instructions. You can always come here to this place of relaxation any time you want. Use this tool for yourself. Use it often. It is your gift. It is within you. You are an amazing human being. You are powerful. You can and will achieve whatever you desire. Let's now have a moment of silence so you can go within yourself and experience yourself more completely.

Download your scripts at www.VictoriaMGallagher.com/wlpbook

Trance Termination Scripts

Drift off or Wake up

Now if it's time for sleep you allow yourself to drift off into dreamy drowsy deep sleep and you will simply bypass any of the remaining suggestions for waking. If it's time for you to come back to full waking consciousness, you will do so at the count of 5, feeling relaxed and well rested, like you are waking up from a nice long nap. If you are ready to come back, you'll come up slowly and gently at the count of 5.

Number one. You are beginning to feel your body where it has been resting so still and quiet and notice the blood flow begin to pick up its pace a little, perhaps by noticing a tingling in your fingers, your head or your toes. Number two. Waking up even more. Good feel your body emerging from its restful state into a wakeful energetic state. Good and three. That's right you are ready to be wakeful, so breathe in the wakeful energy and breathe out any feelings of being tired.

Notice how good it feels to become wakeful again. Number four, almost there. You can now move your arms and your legs, wiggle your fingers and toes and stre-e-e-tch out your torso so. Good. Five. Eyes wide open. You are fully alert and ready to be responsive and energetic. You have all your energy and you perfectly wide awake.

(Give the client a little time to get coherent again and assess their experience.)

(Take notes)

Download your scripts at www.VictoriaMGallagher.com/wlpbook

Waking on the Count of 5

I will now count from 1 to 5. You may continue to remain in this relaxed state for as long as you like and bypass my suggestions if you want to stay in this state. Or on the count of 5, you will be wide awake, alert and ready to continue on with your day. Once again, you will remain relaxed for as long as you like, you will come back naturally and easily on your own and should you drift off to sleep, you will sleep soundly and deeply and wake up feeling refreshed and energized.

If it's time for you to come back, you will be fully awake by the count of five. Number 1, notice the atmosphere in the room you're in. 2... Coming back more and more, feeling your body now... Number 3... wakeful energy moving through your entire body... Number 4... breathing in wakeful energy... waking you up completely, clearing your mind, and filling your body with waking energy. Number 5... you are wide awake and full of energy. Open your eyes and come fully back to waking consciousness.

Download your scripts at www.VictoriaMGallagher.com/wlpbook

Final Thoughts

Now that you've read through the entire 12-Week Hypnosis Program you are ready to apply what you've learned in either your own life or to help inspire the lives of others who need you to guide them on their journey toward a healthier lifestyle.

Feel free to take what you have learned here and design your own custom program that works best for you. There are limitless approaches to working with these sessions and hypnotherapy scripts contained in this manual. Tailor it to best serve you and your unique clients.

You may find that you want to swap sessions with some other therapeutic modality you specialize in. For example, perhaps you do energy work, such as EFT. You might customize the program into a 6-week program, trimming the pieces which your client already has a good handle on. Or you might find your client wants to work with you biweekly, and you could include email support, Facebook group support, a weekly 15-minute emergency call and turn it into a 6-month program.

This could also be turned into a class or a seminar or weekly group coaching. The possibilities are endless!

Understand that this book is only a model based on what has worked for me in my own life and what I use when dealing with weight loss clients. I believe there needs to be a balance between each of these twelve steps. Where you begin your unique journey may differ from the exact routine I have laid out. Feel free to modify it to best fit your own needs or the needs of your client.

Regardless of which way you use this material, realize that by your commitment to being consistent with any of the approaches outlined here, you are going to create favorable results.

If you would like to obtain additional hypnosis scripts to compliment this program, I have written hundreds of amazing hypnosis scripts and you will find those at https://www.hyptalk.com

About the Author

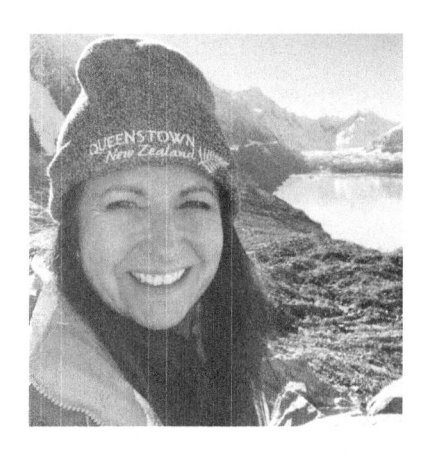

Victoria Gallagher is a worldwide leader in Hypnotherapy, a best-selling author, international speaker, life success coach, and renowned authority on the law of attraction.

Since 1999, Victoria has influenced the lives of hundreds of thousands of people. As creator of a vast library of unique and powerful personal development programs, she helps people change limiting beliefs and achieve their dreams. Her work receives countless high reviews on her popular website Hyptalk.com, which attests to the effectiveness of these programs.

Victoria's work caught the interest of ABC's 20/20 in July 2013, where she was interviewed by Dan Harris in an episode entitled

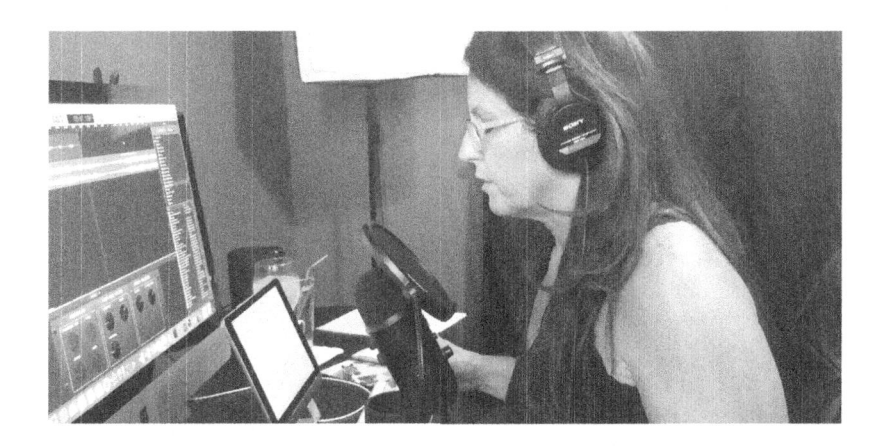

"Got Luck?" She's also been a featured guest on dozens of other radio and online talk shows.

As a tireless personal growth enthusiast herself, Victoria hosts two popular weekly Law of Attraction talk shows, "Law of Attraction Live" and her podcast called "The Power of Your Mind." Both shows feature industry experts and is a powerful platform where you get high value tips and strategies, useful in your everyday life.

Victoria lives an adventurous dream lifestyle in the hiking mecca and scenic town of Cave Creek, Arizona. When she and her soulmate and husband of 11 years, Steve Gallagher, are not busy travelling the world, they spend their free time playing around with their three beautiful housecats, Emerald, Sebastian and Velvet.

Learn more about Victoria Gallagher by visiting:

VictoriaMGallagher.com.

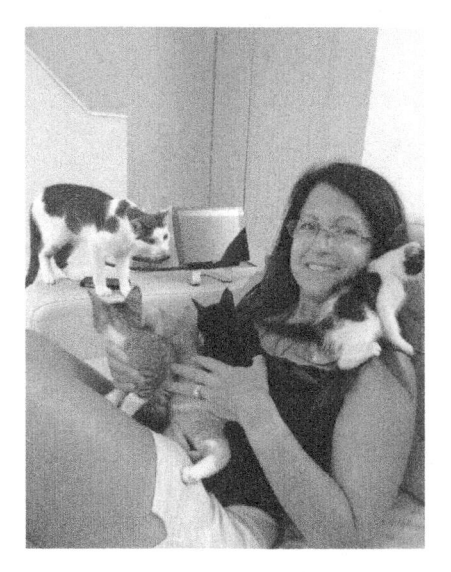